# Helping Young Children Ages 3–8

# Navigate Life Between Two Homes

## Answering the Hard Questions With Compassion and Clarity

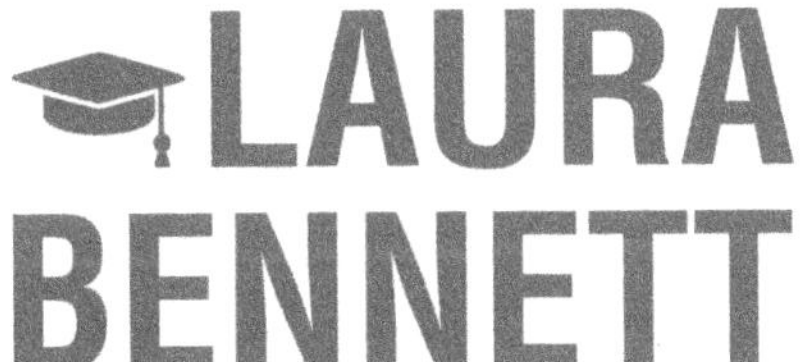

**The Steady Ground Series**

## Guidance for Parents Supporting Young Children Ages 3–8 Through Change

The Steady Ground Series offers calm, developmentally informed guidance for parents navigating family change while raising young children. Each volume focuses on answering the hard questions children ask—or express through behavior—during times of disruption, using language that supports emotional safety, trust, and resilience.

These books are grounded in early childhood development and trauma-informed understanding. They are written for parents who want to respond with steadiness, clarity, and care—even when circumstances feel uncertain.

Children do not need perfect circumstances. They need at least one steady adult who understands what they are feeling.

## Books in the Series

### Talking to Young Children Ages 3–8 About Divorce and Parental Addiction: Answering the Hard Questions with Compassion and Clarity

### Helping Young Children Ages 3–8 Navigate Life Between Two Homes: Answering the Hard Questions with Compassion and Clarity

## Who This Book Is For

This book is for parents of young children navigating life between two homes.

It is for those raising children ages three through eight during divorce or separation—especially when transitions feel harder than expected. It is for parents who notice meltdowns before exchanges, clinginess at bedtime, or quiet withdrawal that doesn't quite make sense.

It is for those who want to respond with steadiness even when co-parenting feels complicated. It is for caregivers supporting sensitive, anxious, or neurodivergent children who experience change intensely.

You do not need to have every answer. You do not need perfect coordination between households. You only need the willingness to understand what moving between two homes feels like from your child's perspective.

This book offers guidance for building emotional safety, predictability, and trust—one steady interaction at a time.

# TABLE OF CONTENTS

# INTRODUCTION

When a family separates and young children begin moving between two homes, parents often focus first on the logistics—who picks up when, what goes in the backpack, how to manage the calendar. But beneath those practical details lies a deeper question that keeps parents awake at night: Is *my child okay?* The answer depends less on perfect schedules or cooperative shared parenting than on something more fundamental—whether children feel emotionally safe as they navigate their new reality.

That emotional security—not logistics—is the heart of this book. It explores what moving between homes actually feels like to young children ages three through eight, whose understanding of time, memory, and belonging differs profoundly from adult experience. A four-year-old doesn't think about custody arrangements or fair division of parenting time. She thinks about whether Mommy will still be there when she comes back. Can her stuffed rabbit come with her? And why does her tummy hurt every Sunday afternoon? Similarly, a seven-year-old doesn't process separation through logic or legal frameworks. He experiences it through his nervous system—the tightness in his chest when he hears the car pull up, the way his body remembers that transitions feel hard even when he can't explain why.

Understanding these internal experiences changes everything about how parents can support their children. When parents recognize that a meltdown before pickup isn't manipulation but communication about overwhelming feelings, they can respond with steadiness rather than frustration. A child's clinginess signals a need for reassurance about connection rather than a problem to fix, allowing parents to offer comfort that actually helps. This child development perspective—seeing transitions through the child's emotional reality first—forms the foundation of every strategy in this book.

The guidance offered here acknowledges something many parenting books sidestep: co-parenting after separation is often messy, strained, and far from the collaborative ideal we imagine. Many of you reading these pages are navigating high-conflict situations where the other parent undermines routines, dismisses concerns, or actively creates instability. Some co-parent with former partners navigating addiction recovery or mental health conditions. Others face the exhausting reality of trying to protect their child from conflict while maintaining boundaries with someone who refuses to communicate constructively. You don't need an ideal co-parenting relationship for this book to work. Instead, it focuses relentlessly on what individual parents can control—their own responses, the routines and emotional anchors they create in their household, and the specific ways they talk to and support their child regardless of what happens elsewhere.

Special attention throughout these chapters goes to neurodivergent kids — those with ADHD, autism spectrum differences, dyslexia, and sensory processing differences—who often experience transitions with greater intensity than neurotypical peers. These children need adapted strategies that honor how their brains and nervous systems process change, manage executive functioning challenges, regulate sensory input, and handle emotional overwhelm. Rather than treating neurodivergent needs as an afterthought, I've integrated specific adaptations into each major concept. If you've been desperately seeking guidance that actually fits your child's experience, this book is for you.

You'll find concrete communication scripts and step-by-step transition routines. You'll discover self-regulation strategies for both children and adults, plus frameworks for building consistency even when the other household operates completely differently. Throughout this book, I'll remind you that you don't need to be perfect to help your child feel secure. What matters most? Showing up with steadiness, offering age-appropriate reassurance, and creating pockets of predictability that help young children develop the internal resilience to navigate an imperfect situation. That work begins with understanding what two homes actually feel like—and that's where this book starts.

Some of the ideas you encounter in this book will return in different forms. That repetition is intentional. When families are under stress, clarity comes not from hearing something once, but from revisiting what matters in moments when you need it most.

## CHAPTER 1

# <u>What Two Homes Feels Like</u>
## Understanding Transitions from Your Young Child's Perspective

A four-year-old stands at the door with her backpack, looking back at her mother's face, then forward toward her father's car. She doesn't have the words yet to say what this moment feels like—the pull between two places she loves, the confusion about where "home" is, the worry that leaving one parent might somehow make them disappear.

This is the reality that countless young children navigate every week, sometimes every few days—a journey between worlds that adults often reduce to logistics while children experience it as something far more profound. What children experience, though, goes far deeper than these logistics suggest. They're learning to exist in a world that has fundamentally changed shape, where the people they love most no longer share the same space, where "going home" has become a complicated concept rather than a simple destination.

If you're reading this, you're likely living inside that complexity right now. You might be watching your child cling to your leg at pickup time, or melt down over packing their favorite stuffed animal, or go suddenly quiet when it's time to leave for their other parent's house. You might be wondering if these behaviors mean something is deeply wrong, if you're failing them somehow, or if the back-and-forth between homes is causing damage you can't undo. You might be exhausted from trying to coordinate with a former partner who won't cooperate, or concerned by how intensely your sensitive or neurodivergent child struggles with change, or simply overwhelmed by the weight of trying to make a difficult situation feel safe for your young child.

This chapter exists to help you understand what your child is actually experiencing during these transitions—not what the parenting plan says should happen, but what it genuinely feels like inside a young child's body and mind to move between two homes. When you understand that your three-year-old's meltdown isn't manipulation but communication, that your six-year-old's sudden clinginess reflects their developmental understanding of separation, that your eight-year-old's withdrawal might be their way of managing emotional overload, you can respond with steadiness instead of panic. You can offer what they actually need rather than what you fear you're supposed to provide.

Throughout this chapter, you'll learn how children ages three through eight experience time, memory, attachment, and change differently than adults do—and why those differences make transitions between homes feel so much bigger and more frightening than we might assume. You'll discover what various transition behaviors are really communicating, including the specific ways neurodivergent children with ADHD, autism, or sensory sensitivities experience these moments with heightened intensity. You'll begin to recognize the invisible emotional load your child carries between homes—the questions they don't ask, the worries they can't name, the loyalty conflicts they feel but can't articulate.

Most importantly, you'll start building your foundation as being the stable parent—the one who can hold calm even when your other parent creates chaos, who can offer predictability even when you can't control what happens at the other house, who can be the secure base your child needs even on days when you feel anything but secure yourself.

You don't need to be perfect at this. You don't need your ex-partner's cooperation to make a meaningful difference. You don't need to have all the answers or get every transition exactly right. What you need is understanding—of what your child is experiencing, what they need from you, and what you can actually control. That understanding starts here, with seeing these everyday moments of transition through your child's eyes rather than through the lens of adult logistics or conflict. When you can hold that perspective, everything else becomes clearer.

## How Young Children Experience Time and Separation Differently Than Adults

When a parent says, "I'll see you in three days," an adult brain translates this into a manageable chunk of time—seventy-two hours that can be measured, anticipated, and contextualized within a larger timeline. A five-year-old hears the same words and experiences something entirely different. For young children, particularly those under age seven, time doesn't flow as an objective, measurable river. Instead, it stretches and compresses based on what fills it, how it feels, and how much attention they're paying to its passage.

Research from developmental psychologists at Eötvös Loránd University demonstrates that children aged four and five judge time primarily through event density rather than absolute duration. In their studies, preschoolers consistently perceived eventful periods as longer than uneventful ones of identical clock time, while adults showed the opposite pattern. This fundamental difference means that when a child waits for a parent during a separation, an uneventful afternoon can feel interminable—not because they're being dramatic, but because their developing brains genuinely process that waiting time as extended and slow.

This changes around age seven, when children start developing what researchers call a symbolic representation of time—the ability to understand time as something that flows uniformly regardless of what's happening within it. Before this developmental milestone, a three-year-old waiting two hours for pickup experiences those hours through the lens of what fills them: the number of activities, the emotional intensity, the novelty of the experience. If those hours are spent anxiously watching for a parent's car, checking the window repeatedly, asking caregivers when Mommy is coming, the time genuinely feels longer than two hours spent absorbed in play.

Emotional arousal compounds this distortion. Studies by developmental researcher Sylvie Droit-Volet show that emotional stimuli—particularly anxiety-provoking ones—speed up children's internal clocks, making durations feel extended. When a child feels worried or uncertain during a transition, their perception of time literally lengthens. The fifteen-minute car ride to the other parent's house, filled with nervous anticipation, registers as significantly longer than the same fifteen minutes spent in calm, familiar routine.

Little ones also experience separations as proportionally larger chunks of their lived experience than adults do. A weekend away from one parent represents a much larger fraction of a four-year-old's conscious memory than it does for a thirty-five-year-old. This proportional difference intensifies the subjective weight of separation, making what feels like a brief custody exchange to an adult feel like a significant absence to a child.

For neurodivergent children, these perception of time challenges often intensify. Children with ADHD may struggle even more with estimating duration and waiting through uneventful periods, as their attention systems make it harder to track time's passage consistently. Autistic children, who often rely heavily on predictable sequences and concrete markers, may experience particular distress when time feels elastic or uncertain. A child who needs to know exactly when something will happen cannot easily hold "in a few days" as a meaningful anchor when their brain doesn't yet process time as uniformly flowing.

The practical implication for parents navigating moving between homes is profound: when your child asks, "When will I see you again?" and you answer "Thursday," you're offering information that may not translate into the reassurance you intend. Their question isn't really about the day of the week—it's about whether the separation will feel endless, whether you'll still be there when they return, whether the waiting will be bearable. Understanding this gap between adult time and child time allows parents to offer what children actually need: concrete markers, emotional reassurance, and strategies that help make waiting time feel less empty and frightening, rather than just calendar information that their developing brains can't yet fully process.

## What Transition Behaviors Are Really Communicating: Decoding Clinginess, Meltdowns, and Withdrawal

When a seven-year-old suddenly refuses to pack her backpack the morning of a transition, or a four-year-old melts down in the driveway during pickup, or a six-year-old goes silent and withdrawn after returning from the other parent's house, these behaviors are not random acts of defiance. They are communication—often the most honest communication a child can offer about what's happening inside their body and mind during a moment that feels too big to manage.

Young children lack both the vocabulary and the cognitive development to articulate complex emotional states. They cannot say "I'm experiencing anticipatory anxiety about this transition because it activates my attachment system and makes me worry about whether you'll still be here when I come back." Instead, they cling to your leg. They cannot explain "I'm emotionally flooded and my nervous system is overwhelmed by the competing demands of loving both of you while feeling like I have to choose." Instead, they have a meltdown. They cannot articulate "I feel unsafe expressing my real feelings because I'm afraid it will hurt you or cause more conflict." Instead, they withdraw into silence.

To decode what these behaviors actually communicate, parents must look beneath the surface action to the underlying need or emotional state driving it. Clinginess, for instance, typically signals separation anxiety—the child's fear that separation might be permanent or that the relationship with the departing parent is at risk. Research from developmental attachment studies demonstrates that young children's protest behaviors during separation reflect their need for reassurance about the caregiver's availability and responsiveness, not an attempt to manipulate or control the situation. When a three-year-old wraps both arms around your waist and refuses to let go at drop-off, she's asking a question her words cannot form: "Will you still be mine when I come back? Will leaving you make you disappear?"

Meltdowns communicate something different—they signal that the child's capacity for managing emotions has been exceeded. Young children's prefrontal cortex, the brain region responsible for managing big emotions and inhibiting impulses, remains under development throughout early childhood. When the emotional demand of a transition overwhelms this developing system, a meltdown is the neurological result, not a behavioral choice. The bigger the meltdown, often the bigger the internal experience—how frightening the transition feels, how uncertain the child is about what comes next, how much emotional work they've been doing to hold themselves together.

Withdrawal represents perhaps the most concerning communication because it often goes unnoticed or gets mistaken for adjustment. When a child becomes quiet, compliant, and emotionally flat around moving between homes, they may be signaling that their system has moved into a protective shutdown state. Withdrawal can indicate that the child has learned their feelings are not safe to express—perhaps because previous expressions led to parental distress, conflict between parents, or messages that the child should "be brave" or "not make this harder." It can also reflect emotional exhaustion, where the child simply has no more capacity to process or express what they're experiencing.

For neurodivergent children, these communication patterns often intensify or manifest differently. A child with ADHD may experience emotional dysregulation more intensely and recover more slowly, making meltdowns more frequent and prolonged. A child with autism may withdraw not only from emotional overwhelm but also from sensory overload during the physical transition itself—the car ride, the different smells and sounds of the other home, the unpredictability of the schedule. A highly sensitive child may absorb and internalize parental tension during handoffs, leading to behaviors that emerge hours later, seemingly disconnected from the transition itself.

The essential insight for parents is this: these behaviors are not problems to eliminate but messages to decode. When parents can receive clinginess, meltdowns, and withdrawal as communication rather than defiance, they can respond to the actual need underneath—offering reassurance for separation anxiety, co-regulation support for overwhelm, and explicit safety for emotional expression.

## The Neurodivergent Child's Experience: Why ADHD, Autism, and Sensory Sensitivities Intensify Transition Stress

For neurodivergent children—those with ADHD, autism spectrum differences, or sensory processing sensitivities—the stress of transitions between homes doesn't just feel harder. It registers neurologically as a fundamentally different and more overwhelming experience than it does for neurotypical peers. Understanding why requires looking at how these children's brains and nervous systems process change, predictability, sensory input, and emotional regulation.

Children with ADHD face particular challenges with transitions because of differences in executive function—the brain's ability to shift gears, plan ahead, manage time, and regulate emotional responses to change. Research on executive function in ADHD demonstrates that these children struggle significantly more than neurotypical peers with task-switching and adapting to new contexts. When a child with ADHD needs to pack a bag, remember what goes to which house, shift from one parent's routine to another's, and manage the emotional weight of saying goodbye, they're being asked to coordinate multiple executive function demands simultaneously—precisely the area where their brain development creates the most difficulty. The result isn't willful resistance or defiance; it's genuine neurological overwhelm that can show up as meltdowns, avoidance, or complete shutdown when transition time approaches.

The ADHD brain also experiences emotional regulation differently. Research shows that children with ADHD often experience emotions more intensely and have greater difficulty managing their responses—what researchers call emotional impulsivity. During transitions, this means that anxiety, sadness, or frustration about leaving one parent doesn't just feel uncomfortable—it floods the system with an intensity that can feel unbearable. The emotional recovery time after a difficult transition also extends longer for children with ADHD, meaning they may still be dysregulated hours after arriving at the other home, even when the transition itself appeared to go smoothly.

Autistic children face a different but equally significant set of challenges rooted in their need for predictability and sameness. Research on autism consistently shows that unexpected changes or disruptions to established routines trigger stronger stress responses in autistic children than in neurotypical children. For an autistic child, each home represents a complex sensory and social environment with specific rules, expectations, sounds, smells, textures, and interpersonal dynamics. Moving between these environments requires constant recalibration—learning which behaviors are expected here versus there, which sensory inputs to prepare for, which social scripts apply in this context. This cognitive and sensory labor is exhausting, and when the two homes operate with different routines or expectations, the child must hold two separate behavioral maps in mind and switch between them repeatedly.

Sensory processing differences compound this challenge across both ADHD and autism, as well as for children with sensory processing disorder. Different homes inevitably contain different sensory environments—lighting, noise levels, food textures, clothing options, bedding materials, even the smell of laundry detergent. For children with sensory sensitivities, these differences aren't minor preferences—they're neurological experiences that can range from uncomfortable to genuinely distressing. A child who is sensitive to sound may find one parent's home overwhelming due to traffic noise or a louder household, while the other home feels calmer. A child with tactile sensitivities may struggle with different bedding or clothing options at each house, making basic comfort harder to achieve.

Together, these neurological differences mean that neurodivergent children carry a significantly heavier cognitive, sensory, and emotional load during transitions than neurotypical children do. They're not being more challenging—they're managing genuinely more challenging internal experiences. When parents understand this distinction, they can respond to transition struggles with the accommodations and support these children actually need rather than with frustration about behaviors that look like resistance but are actually communication about overwhelm.

## The Invisible Emotional Load: What Children Carry Between Homes That Parents Don't Always See

Beyond the visible behaviors—the tears at drop-off, the backpack left behind, the meltdown over mismatched socks—young children carry an emotional weight between homes that parents rarely see and children rarely name. This hidden emotional burden consists of worries too complex to articulate, questions too scary to ask out loud. Emotional labor that no three-year-old should have to manage but many do anyway.

A five-year-old wonders silently whether mentioning Dad's new apartment will make Mom sad. So she edits her stories carefully, leaving out half of what happened during her weekend away.

A seven-year-old packs his favorite stuffed animal, then unpacks it, then packs it again, paralyzed by the impossible choice of which parent gets to see him sleep with it tonight.

A six-year-old watches her mother's face during pickup, scanning for signs of tension or sadness. She adjusts her own enthusiasm accordingly—learning to perform "okayness" to protect the parent she's leaving behind.

This emotional labor mirrors what researchers call the invisible load adults carry in managing family life—the mental planning, anticipatory work, and emotion regulation that happens beneath the surface of visible tasks.

Studies on parental emotional labor demonstrate that this cognitive and emotional burden includes anticipating needs, managing interpersonal dynamics, and maintaining others' emotional comfort, work that becomes visible only when it's not done.

Young children in two-home families perform a developmentally inappropriate version of this same labor: they anticipate parental reactions, manage loyalty conflicts, suppress feelings that might create tension.

They work constantly to reconcile two different sets of expectations, routines, and emotional climates.

The cognitive demand alone is significant. Children must remember which rules apply in which home—bedtime at seven-thirty here, eight-thirty there; screen time allowed on weekends at Dad's but not at Mom's.

Different expectations about homework, chores, and manners.

They must track which belongings live where, which topics are safe to discuss with which parent, which version of family stories matches which household's narrative.

This mental load of code-switching between homes requires executive function skills that are still developing in children ages three through eight, creating exhaustion that parents often mistake for moodiness or resistance.

The emotional component runs even deeper.

Children carry unspoken questions that feel too dangerous to voice:

Is the divorce my fault?

Will you stop loving me if I love my other parent too much?

What happens if I like it better at one house?

If I'm happy here, does that hurt the parent I just left?

We know from research on children's emotional development that young children are highly attuned to parental emotional states and will suppress their own feelings to avoid causing distress to caregivers they depend on for safety.

In two-home situations, this protective instinct doubles—children monitor and manage their emotional expression to avoid hurting either parent, creating an internal pressure that has nowhere to go.

For neurodivergent children, this invisible load intensifies significantly.

A child with ADHD may struggle intensely with the executive function demands of tracking different rules and belongings across homes, experiencing this cognitive labor as overwhelming rather than just difficult.

An autistic child may carry the additional burden of masking—suppressing their authentic responses and needs to fit different social expectations in each environment—which research shows leads to significant emotional exhaustion and increased anxiety over time.

Highly sensitive children absorb parental tension during moving between homes like emotional sponges, carrying worry about their parents' wellbeing that they cannot name or release.

Parents cannot eliminate this invisible load entirely—the reality of two homes creates inherent complexity.

But recognizing that it exists, that children are working hard internally even when they appear fine externally, allows parents to respond with the reassurance, explicit permission, and emotional safety that lightens what children carry alone in silence.


## Building Your Foundation as the Steady Parent: What You Can Control When Co-Parenting Is Hard

When everything about co-parenting feels chaotic and beyond your influence, the question that matters most is deceptively simple: what can you actually control?

The answer is both smaller and more powerful than most parents realize.

You cannot control your former partner's choices, their emotional state, their parenting approach, or how they speak about you to your child.

You cannot control whether they follow through on agreements, maintain consistent routines, or prioritize your child's needs over their own grievances.

In high-conflict situations, you may not even be able to control the basic logistics of pickups and drop-offs without tension or last-minute changes.

But you can control yourself.

You can control your own nervous system, your responses, your home environment, and the emotional climate you create during your parenting time. This distinction—between what lies outside your sphere of influence and what sits squarely within it—becomes the foundation of being the steady parent your child needs.

Research on parental influence during family transitions demonstrates that children's adjustment to divorce depends less on whether both parents cooperate smoothly and more on whether at least one parent provides consistent emotional safety and regulation.

Studies from developmental psychology show that when one parent remains predictable, emotionally available, and calm despite ongoing conflict, children develop secure attachment and resilience even when the other household remains chaotic or unpredictable. Your steadiness matters more than achieving perfect co-parenting harmony.

## Your Emotional Regulation Is Your Primary Tool

The most important element within your control is your own emotional state, particularly during the charged moments of transitions. Young children are neurologically wired to read parental emotional cues as information about safety. When you arrive at pickup visibly tense, angry, or anxious—even if you say nothing—your child's nervous system registers threat. When you maintain calm, your child's developing stress response system learns that transitions, while difficult, are manageable.

This does not mean performing fake cheerfulness or suppressing legitimate feelings.

It means developing the capacity to notice your own dysregulation—the tight chest, the racing thoughts, the urge to respond defensively to your co-parent's latest provocation—and choosing to pause rather than react.

Techniques such as deep breathing before arrivals, taking a moment in the car to ground yourself, or having a trusted friend on standby for post-transition processing all serve the same purpose: they help you arrive regulated so your child can borrow your calm.

For parents of neurodivergent children, this regulation becomes even more critical.

Children with ADHD or autism are particularly sensitive to environmental stress and parental emotional states. They may absorb your tension and mirror it back as dysregulation hours later, seemingly disconnected from the transition itself. When you manage your own nervous system, you provide the co-regulation scaffold these children need to manage theirs.

## What You Say and Don't Say About the Other Parent

You control completely what you communicate to your child about their other parent.

This includes explicit statements, but also tone, facial expressions when the other parent's name comes up, and the stories you tell about why the family changed.

Research consistently shows that children who are shielded from negative commentary about either parent—even when that commentary feels justified—experience less anxiety, fewer loyalty conflicts, and healthier long-term adjustment.

This boundary protects your child, not your co-parent.

When your seven-year-old mentions something that happened at Dad's house and you respond with warmth rather than criticism, you're teaching her that loving both parents is safe.

When your five-year-old asks why you don't live together anymore and you offer a simple, blame-free explanation, you're lifting the invisible burden of choosing sides.

## The Consistency of Your Home Environment

Within your own household, you have complete authority over routines, rules, and the physical environment. This control is your most tangible tool for creating security. Consistent bedtimes, predictable mealtimes, familiar rituals around homework or bath time—these patterns become anchors that help children feel safe even when everything else feels uncertain.

You cannot make the other household match yours, and trying to enforce consistency across both homes when your co-parent won't cooperate is an exercise in frustration. But you can make your home reliably, predictably yours. That reliability alone provides enormous developmental benefit.

The four-year-old standing at the door with her backpack, looking between her mother's face and her father's car, is doing something extraordinary.

She's holding two worlds in her small body, navigating an emotional complexity that most adults would struggle to manage, and doing it without the language, cognitive development, or life experience to make sense of what she's feeling.

She's asking questions she cannot voice, carrying worries she cannot name, and working harder than anyone around her may realize to love both parents without betraying either one.

Understanding what moving between homes feel like from your child's perspective changes everything about how you respond to them.

When you recognize that your three-year-old's meltdown isn't manipulation but communication about overwhelm, that your six-year-old's clinginess reflects separation anxiety rather than defiance, that your eight-year-old's withdrawal signals emotional exhaustion rather than adjustment, you can meet these behaviors with what they actually need: reassurance, co-regulation, and the steady presence of a parent who isn't frightened by big feelings.

The developmental realities explored in this chapter—how young children experience time as elastic rather than linear, how their brains process separation as proportionally larger than adults do, how their limited executive functioning makes the cognitive demands of two homes genuinely overwhelming—are not obstacles to overcome but truths to honor.

Your child isn't being difficult when they struggle with transitions. They're managing a genuinely difficult internal experience with a brain that's still learning how to regulate emotions, track time, and hold complexity.

For neurodivergent children, these challenges intensify in specific, predictable ways that require specialized understanding and support.

The child with ADHD who melts down every time packing begins isn't being oppositional—their executive function differences make task-switching and emotional regulation neurologically harder.

The autistic child who scripts the same phrases repeatedly on transition days isn't being rigid—they're using language to create predictability in a moment that feels chaotic.

The highly sensitive child who goes quiet after pickup isn't fine—they're overwhelmed by sensory and emotional input they cannot yet process.

When parents understand these neurological differences, they can respond with accommodations rather than frustration, support rather than correction.

Perhaps most importantly, this chapter establishes what sits within your control when so much feels chaotic and uncertain. You cannot change your other parent's choices, eliminate the complexity of two homes, or make transitions easy.

But you can control your own emotional regulation during handoffs, the consistency and predictability of your household routines, what you say and don't say about the other parent. The emotional climate you create during your parenting time.

Research consistently demonstrates that children develop resilience and secure attachment when at least one parent provides steady, emotionally available care—even when the other household remains unpredictable or the co-parenting relationship stays conflicted.

Your steadiness matters more than perfection. Your regulation matters more than having all the answers. Your willingness to see transitions through your child's eyes rather than through the lens of adult logistics or conflict creates the foundation for everything that follows in this book.

The chapters ahead will build on this foundation with specific strategies, scripts, and approaches for supporting your child before, during, and after transitions.

You'll learn what to say when your child asks hard questions, how to create routines that work even without co-parent cooperation, and how to recognize when your child needs additional support.

But all of those practical tools rest on the understanding you've gained here: that your child's experience of moving between homes is profound, complex, and deserving of your compassionate attention—and that you have more power to support them through it than you might have believed possible.

# Reading the Signs
## Recognizing Dysregulation and Anxiety in Children Ages 3-8 During Custody Changes

Your six-year-old who usually loves bedtime stories suddenly refuses to settle down on nights before custody exchanges, bouncing off the walls until exhaustion takes over.

Your three-year-old, who was finally potty trained, starts having accidents again every time she returns from her other parent's house.

These moments naturally raise important questions: Is this normal adjustment, or is something deeper going on? How do you know when your child needs more support, and what exactly are you looking for?

Understanding what to look for begins with an important truth: nervous system overwhelm and anxiety in young children don't always look the way parents expect them to.

We often imagine tears and tantrums, but distress in children ages three through eight shows up in dozens of quieter, more confusing ways—bedwetting, stomachaches, sudden defiance, withdrawal, sleep disruption, or that frantic, bouncing energy that seems to come from nowhere.

For neurologically different children, the signs can be even harder to read because their baseline behaviors already differ from neurotypical peers, and their nervous systems respond to transition stress with unique intensity.

This chapter teaches you to become a skilled observer of your own child's specific signals. You'll learn what dysregulation actually means in early childhood development—not misbehavior or manipulation, but a nervous system overwhelmed by more than it can process.

You'll discover how anxiety manifests differently at age three versus age seven, why some children's distress goes completely underground, and how ADHD, autism, sensory processing differences, and high sensitivity change what struggling looks like from the outside.

Understanding these signs matters because you cannot support what you cannot see.

When you recognize that your five-year-old's sudden pickiness about food on transition days is actually an anxiety response, you can offer regulation support instead of fighting about vegetables.

When you notice that your seven-year-old gets quieter and more compliant after visits to her dad's house—performing okayness rather than feeling it—you can create space for her real feelings instead of assuming she's fine.

Recognition is the first step toward responsive support.

This chapter also addresses a fear many parents carry: that noticing these signs means you're failing, that your child's dysregulation is evidence that the divorce is damaging them beyond repair, or that you should somehow be able to prevent all distress.

The reality is gentler and more hopeful.

Nervous System Overwhelm during major life transitions is normal, expected, and not a sign of permanent harm. What matters most is not whether your child shows signs of stress—most children living between two homes will at some point—but whether they have a parent who notices, responds with steadiness, and helps them return to regulation over time.

You'll learn to track patterns without panic, distinguishing between temporary adjustment responses and signs that your child needs additional professional support. You'll discover simple observation tools that help you understand your child's unique stress signals without turning parenting into constant surveillance.

And you'll gain clarity about what you can do with this information—how recognizing dysregulation empowers you to respond proactively with the trauma-informed strategies that follow in later chapters.

For parents navigating high-conflict co-parenting, this chapter acknowledges a painful reality: you may be the only one noticing or responding to your child's distress signals. Your co-parent may dismiss concerns, blame you for creating problems, or simply not have the capacity to see what you're seeing.

This chapter focuses on what you can observe and respond to within your own time with your child, building your confidence as the steady, attuned parent who helps your child make sense of what their body and emotions are trying to tell them.

## The Body Speaks First: Physical Signs of Nervous System Overwhelm in Young Children (Sleep Disruption, Appetite Changes, Toileting Regression, Stomachaches)

Understanding how children communicate distress begins with a developmental reality: before young children have the language to say, "I'm anxious about going to Dad's house" or "I feel scared when things keep changing," their bodies speak for them. Physical symptoms are often the first and clearest signals that a child is struggling with the stress of custody changes—and for parents trying to decode what their child needs, these bodily signs provide essential information that words cannot yet convey.

Sleep disruption stands as one of the most common physical indicators of nervous system overwhelm during custody changes. A child who previously slept through the night may suddenly resist bedtime, experience frequent nightmares, or wake repeatedly calling for a parent. These patterns often intensify on nights before custody exchanges or immediately following a return from the other home.

The disruption reflects the child's nervous system remaining in a state of heightened alertness, unable to relax into the deep rest that requires feeling fundamentally safe.

For neurodivergent children, particularly those with ADHD or autism who already experience sleep challenges, custody changes can compound existing difficulties. An autistic child's carefully constructed bedtime routine may be impossible to replicate across two homes, leaving their body unable to recognize the safety signals needed for sleep. A child with ADHD may find their already-active mind racing with questions and worries about the upcoming transition, their planning and organizing abilities too overwhelmed to initiate the calming sequence that leads to rest.

Appetite changes provide another window into a child's internal state. Some children lose interest in food entirely during high-stress periods, picking at meals or complaining that their stomach feels funny. Others eat significantly more than usual, seeking comfort and control through food when other aspects of life feel unpredictable.

Weight fluctuations, sudden pickiness about previously accepted foods, or complaints of nausea around mealtimes all signal that the child's digestive system is responding to emotional distress. The gut-brain connection in young children is particularly strong—anxiety literally affects their ability to feel hungry, digest food comfortably, or enjoy eating.

Highly sensitive children may become acutely aware of textures, temperatures, and flavors during stressful periods, rejecting foods that feel overwhelming to their heightened sensory systems.

Toileting regression represents one of the most distressing physical signs for both children and parents. A child who achieved consistent daytime or nighttime dryness may suddenly begin having accidents again or experiencing bedwetting.

This regression is not willful or manipulative—it reflects a nervous system so overwhelmed that it temporarily loses capacity for skills that require significant self-regulation and body awareness. The shame children feel about these accidents often compounds their distress, creating a cycle where anxiety about toileting leads to more accidents, which increases anxiety further.

For children with developmental differences or those who achieved toileting skills later than peers, regression during custody stress may feel particularly devastating to their sense of competence and growing independence.

Stomachaches and headaches round out the constellation of physical symptoms that signal nervous system overwhelm. These stress-related physical symptoms complaints—real physical sensations generated by emotional distress—appear frequently in young children who lack the developmental capacity to name anxiety, sadness, or fear directly.

A five-year-old cannot always say "I feel anxious about the transition tomorrow," but she can say "my tummy hurts." A seven-year-old may not have words for the loyalty conflict he feels between two homes, but he knows his head pounds on Sunday evenings before the exchange. These complaints deserve to be taken seriously, not dismissed as manipulation or attention-seeking. The pain is genuine, even when medical examination reveals no physical cause.

Recognizing these physical signs allows parents to respond with compassion rather than frustration, understanding that the body is doing exactly what it should do—communicating distress when words are not yet available.

# Behavioral Signals Across Ages 3-8: What Dysregulation Looks Like at Different Developmental Stages

Moving from physical signs to behavioral patterns, it's important to recognize that dysregulation looks remarkably different in a three-year-old than it does in an eight-year-old, not because the underlying distress is less real at any age, but because children's developmental capacities shape how that distress emerges into the world.

Understanding these age-specific patterns helps parents recognize when their child is struggling and respond in ways that match where their child actually is developmentally, rather than where parents wish they could be.

### Ages Three to Four: When the Body Does All the Talking

At three and four, children possess limited language for internal experiences and almost no capacity for abstract thinking about time, change, or family structure. Nervous System Overwhelm at this age shows up almost entirely through the body and through behavior. A three-year-old cannot say "I feel anxious about the transition tomorrow"—instead, she clings to her mother's leg at drop-off, screaming with an intensity that seems disproportionate to the moment. A four-year-old who feels overwhelmed by moving between homes may hit, bite, or throw toys when frustrated, his stress response system flooding with emotion he has no words to contain.

Tantrums at this age become more frequent, longer, and harder to soothe when a child is dysregulated by custody stress. While all preschoolers have tantrums, dysregulated tantrums happen multiple times daily, escalate rapidly from calm to explosive, and resist the usual soothing strategies that previously worked.

Sleep becomes fragile—bedtime suddenly requires an hour of resistance, nightmares increase, or a child who slept independently now refuses to be alone. Toileting regression appears commonly, with previously trained children having frequent accidents or bedwetting that correlates directly with transition days.

For neurodivergent children at this age, dysregulation intensifies existing challenges. A three-year-old autistic child may lose speech entirely during high-stress moments, reverting to nonverbal communication or familiar phrases. A child with sensory processing differences may become unable to tolerate clothing textures, food temperatures, or bath time—ordinary sensory experiences feeling unbearable when their stress response system is already overwhelmed. ADHD traits may amplify, with hyperactivity becoming more intense and impulsivity leading to unsafe behaviors like running away or climbing dangerously.

## Ages Five to Six: When Worry Finds Words

Between five and six, children develop greater emotional vocabulary and begin to express anxiety more directly, though their understanding remains concrete and immediate. Dysregulation at this age often includes verbal expressions of worry—repeated questions about schedules, who will pick them up, whether a parent will be there when they return. A five-year-old might ask the same question ten times in an hour, seeking reassurance that feels impossible to provide adequately.

School becomes a new arena where dysregulation appears. Teachers may report that a previously engaged child now struggles to focus, refuses to participate, or has difficulty following multi-step directions. Social withdrawal emerges—a six-year-old who loved playdates suddenly declines invitations or plays alone at recess. Somatic complaints increase in frequency and specificity: stomachaches before transitions, headaches on Sunday evenings, nausea at breakfast on exchange days.

Defiance and opposition intensify as children this age attempt to exert control over a situation that feels fundamentally uncontrollable. A child may refuse to pack her bag, insist she will not go to the other parent's house, or become rigid about small details—which shoes to wear, which stuffed animal to bring—because these tiny choices represent the only agency she feels she has.

Neurologically Different children at this age may develop rigid routines or rituals to manage anxiety, becoming distressed when these cannot be replicated across homes. An autistic six-year-old might insist on identical bedtime sequences in both houses, melting down when this proves impossible. A child with ADHD may struggle intensely with the planning and organizing abilities demands of packing, transitioning, and remembering belongings across two homes, leading to frequent meltdowns around these tasks.

## Ages Seven to Eight: When Distress Goes Underground

By seven and eight, many children have learned which emotions are acceptable to express and which create tension or conflict.

Dysregulation at this age often becomes more hidden, internalized, and socially masked.

A seven-year-old may appear fine at school and at both parents' homes, then explode in rage over minor frustrations—the emotional suppression finally overwhelming her capacity to hold it together. An eight-year-old might become perfectionistic, anxious about grades, or overly responsible, attempting to control his internal chaos through external achievement.

Social relationships take on greater importance, and dysregulation frequently damages peer connections. Children this age may struggle with emotional reciprocity, becoming clingy with friends or pushing them away with irritability. Academic performance may decline noticeably as concentration suffers and motivation wanes. Some children develop school avoidance, complaining of illness on school mornings or expressing dread about attending.

Lying, stealing, or rule-breaking may emerge as coping mechanisms—a child testing whether rules and relationships are stable, or attempting to exert control through transgression. Sleep disturbances continue but may shift toward difficulty falling asleep due to racing thoughts rather than fear of separation. Appetite changes become more pronounced, with some children eating very little and others seeking comfort through food.

For neurodivergent children, this age brings awareness of their differences from peers, compounding transition stress with social anxiety and identity questions. An eight-year-old with ADHD may recognize that they struggle more than classmates with organization across two homes, leading to shame that intensifies dysregulation. An autistic child may work exhaustingly hard to mask differences at school, then experience significant dysregulation at home where they finally feel safe enough to release the day's accumulated stress.

## When Anxiety Hides: Recognizing Internalized Distress in Quiet, Compliant, or 'Good' Children

Not all distress announces itself loudly. While some children respond to custody transitions with tantrums, defiance, or obvious emotional meltdowns, others turn their anxiety inward, becoming quieter, more compliant, and seemingly easier to manage. These are the children who worry parents in a different way—not because they are falling apart, but because they appear to be holding themselves together too well.

The quiet, compliant child who never complains about transitions, who packs their bag without resistance, who smiles and says they are fine when asked how they feel—this child may actually be carrying significant distress that goes completely unrecognized. Their anxiety does not disappear simply because it remains unexpressed. Instead, it burrows deeper, manifesting in ways that parents and caregivers often miss until the internalized distress reaches a breaking point.

Research on children's responses to divorce and separation confirms that anxiety and depression increase during custody transitions, but these emotional responses do not always present through visible behavioral disruption.

Some children, particularly those with temperaments favoring emotional restraint or those who have learned that expressing distress creates additional tension, channel their anxiety inward rather than outward. Children with certain temperaments may be more likely to internalize distress, though internalization occurs across all genders and temperamental profiles.

Internalized anxiety in young children appears through subtle shifts that require careful observation to detect. Physical complaints without clear medical causes—stomachaches before transitions, headaches on exchange days, unexplained nausea—often signal anxiety expressing itself through the body when a child cannot or will not verbalize emotional distress. These psychosomatic symptoms are genuine physical experiences generated by psychological stress, not manipulation or attention-seeking.

Sleep disturbances provide another window into hidden anxiety. A child may begin having difficulty falling asleep, experience nightmares, or wake frequently during the night without calling out for help. Because these changes can have multiple causes, parents may attribute them to growth phases or minor illness rather than recognizing them as anxiety responses to custody stress.

Emotional withdrawal represents one of the most concerning signs of internalized distress. A previously engaged child becomes quieter, shows less interest in activities they once enjoyed, or displays a flattened emotional range. They may appear sad without being able to articulate why, or they may seem emotionally distant even during moments that would typically bring joy or excitement.

The paradox of the compliant child is that their good behavior may actually mask significant suffering.

A child experiencing anxiety may become even more compliant, attempting to manage their internal chaos through perfect external behavior. They may fear that any misbehavior will result in loss of parental love, or they may believe that their goodness can somehow prevent further family disruption. This heightened alertness to parental expectations requires enormous energy and contributes to their overall anxiety burden, even though it appears externally as model behavior.

Children who internalize distress often struggle to express their emotional experiences verbally. They may lack the language to describe anxiety, or they may fear burdening already-stressed parents with additional worries. A seven-year-old might think, "Mom is already upset about the custody situation; I shouldn't make it worse by telling her I am scared." This self-silencing prevents parents from understanding their child's true emotional state and providing needed support.

Quiet does not mean unreachable. Children who internalize distress can still be deeply supported when parents learn what to look for.

For neurologically different children, internalized anxiety can be particularly difficult to recognize because it may overlap with existing traits. An autistic child's natural preference for routine and emotional reserve may mask growing distress about custody transitions. A child with ADHD who appears hyperactive and unfocused may actually be experiencing significant anxiety that amplifies their existing regulatory challenges, but the anxiety itself remains hidden beneath more visible behaviors.

Recognizing internalized distress requires parents to look beyond surface compliance and good behavior, attending instead to subtle changes in physical health, sleep patterns, emotional engagement, and the quality of a child's presence. The quiet child needs the same attentive support as the child who acts out—perhaps more, because their distress operates in silence.

## The Neurodivergent Difference: How ADHD, Autism, and Sensory Processing Disorders Change What Dysregulation Looks Like

Neurodivergent children experience dysregulation differently than their neurotypical peers, not because their distress is more or less valid, but because their nervous systems process transition stress through distinct neurological pathways. For parents trying to recognize when their ADHD, autistic, or sensory-sensitive child is struggling with custody transitions, understanding these differences becomes essential—what looks like defiance, shutdown, or sensory meltdown is often profound nervous system overwhelm that standard observation frameworks miss entirely.

# ADHD: When Dysregulation Looks Like Chaos

Children with ADHD experience custody changes with intensified emotional volatility and executive function collapse that extends far beyond typical frustration. Research on ADHD and family transitions confirms that these children show rapid mood swings, hyperactivity surges, and impulsivity spikes during periods of routine disruption that persist across multiple days rather than resolving quickly like neurotypical upset. A seven-year-old with ADHD may appear fine during the car ride to the other parent's house, then explode in defiance over a minor request thirty minutes after arrival, his nervous system finally catching up to the transition stress his executive function could not process in real time.

This is not regression or permanent damage. It is a sign your child's system needs longer recovery time than others might.

Dysregulation in ADHD often manifests as constant motion—a child who cannot sit still at meals, who bounces from activity to activity without completing anything, whose body seems to vibrate with unexpressed anxiety. Small routine variances between homes—different bedtimes, varying homework expectations, inconsistent screen time rules—provoke disproportionate emotional floods because the ADHD brain struggles to shift between competing sets of expectations. What parents might interpret as willful defiance is actually a nervous system overwhelmed by the cognitive load of tracking and adapting to two different household systems.

Inattention intensifies during transition periods, with children losing belongings, forgetting instructions immediately after hearing them, or appearing completely unable to focus on tasks they could manage during stable periods. This executive function collapse signals that the child's regulatory capacity is completely consumed by transition stress, leaving nothing available for the ordinary demands of daily life.

## Autism: When Dysregulation Goes Silent

Autistic children's dysregulation during custody changes frequently presents as shutdown rather than meltdown—a complete withdrawal that parents may mistake for calm acceptance. Research on autism and family transitions demonstrates that routine disruption overwhelms autistic children's processing capacity, leading to nonverbal distress, intensified stimming, or rigid adherence to sameness as desperate attempts to maintain internal regulation when external predictability disappears.

Shutdown is a protective response, not disappearance. With safety and predictability, children re-engage.

A five-year-old autistic child may stop speaking entirely during the hours surrounding a custody exchange, reverting to nonverbal communication or scripted phrases from familiar videos. This selective mutism signals profound overwhelm, not willful silence. Stimming behaviors—hand flapping, rocking, repeating sounds—increase in frequency and intensity as the child attempts to self-regulate through sensory input when emotional regulation feels impossible.

Unlike neurotypical children who might verbally express worry about transitions, autistic children often cannot articulate the grief, confusion, or anxiety they experience when family composition shifts. Their distress emerges instead through behavioral rigidity—insisting on identical routines across both homes, melting down over minor environmental differences, or refusing to engage with activities they typically enjoy. These responses reflect genuine trauma-like reactions to disrupted familiarity, not manipulation or stubbornness.

## Sensory Processing Disorders: When Environments Become Unbearable

Children with sensory processing differences experience dysregulation through their bodies' responses to environmental mismatches between homes. A child who thrives in one parent's quiet, dimly lit home may become completely overwhelmed in the other parent's bright, noisy household—not because of preference, but because their nervous system cannot regulate amid sensory input that feels physically painful or chaotic.

Sensory dysregulation appears as tactile defensiveness—suddenly refusing to wear certain clothes, resisting hugs, or reacting with aggression to light touch. It manifests as auditory overload—covering ears, becoming irritable in response to normal household sounds, or shutting down entirely in busy environments. Visual sensitivity intensifies, with children struggling in bright spaces or becoming fixated on visual stimuli as attempts to manage overwhelm.

These physiological responses differ fundamentally from emotional upset in neurotypical children because they originate in the sensory system rather than cognitive processing of the transition itself. A child is not choosing to be difficult about clothing textures—their nervous system genuinely cannot tolerate the sensory input during a period when regulatory capacity is already depleted by custody stress.

Understanding these neurologically different presentations of dysregulation allows parents to respond with appropriate support rather than consequences for behaviors that reflect neurological differences, not defiance.

## Tracking Patterns Without Panic: Creating Simple Observation Tools to Understand Your Child's Unique Stress Signals

Once parents understand what stress response system overwhelm looks like in their child, the next step involves tracking these signals in a way that builds clarity without creating constant surveillance or parental anxiety. The goal is not to document every moment of a child's day or to build evidence for court proceedings, but rather to notice patterns that help parents respond more effectively to their child's unique needs during custody transitions.

Simple observation tools work best when they require minimal time and mental energy to maintain. A parent already managing the emotional labor of co-parenting, work responsibilities, and their own regulation does not need a complex tracking system that adds to their overwhelm. Instead, effective observation focuses on noticing a few key signals consistently over time, creating just enough structure to reveal patterns without turning parenting into data collection.

The most accessible approach involves keeping a brief transition log—a simple notebook, phone note, or calendar entry that captures basic information around custody exchanges. Parents might note the date and time of the transition, one or two observable behaviors in the hours before and after the exchange, and any physical symptoms that appeared. A log entry might read: "Thursday 5pm pickup, refused to pack bag, stomachache at bedtime, woke twice overnight." Another might note: "Sunday return from Dad's, very quiet in car, no appetite at dinner, asked three times if I would be home when he wakes up."

This minimal documentation serves several purposes.

First, it helps parents distinguish between isolated difficult moments and genuine patterns that signal ongoing distress. A single rough transition does not necessarily indicate a problem requiring intervention, but the same constellation of behaviors appearing every week before exchanges reveals a pattern worth addressing.

Second, tracking reduces the cognitive load of trying to remember details across days and weeks, particularly for parents managing ADHD themselves or those whose own stress affects memory and executive function.

Third, simple logs provide concrete information to share with therapists, pediatricians, or other professionals if additional support becomes necessary.

For neurologically different children, observation tools benefit from slightly more specificity about the types of signals most relevant to their particular profile. Parents of children with ADHD might track executive function indicators like difficulty packing, forgetting belongings, or inability to follow multi-step instructions around transitions.

Parents of autistic children might note changes in verbal communication, increases in stimming behaviors, or rigidity about routines. Parents of highly sensitive children might focus on sensory responses—refusal to wear certain clothes, complaints about noise or light, or withdrawal from physical affection.

The key to tracking without panic lies in maintaining emotional neutrality while recording observations. The log is not a place for interpretation, judgment, or catastrophizing—it simply captures what happened. "Refused to go to Dad's, screamed for twenty minutes" is an observation. "Having a complete breakdown because the divorce is ruining him" is panic. The first provides useful information; the second amplifies parental distress without adding clarity.

Parents should review their observations weekly rather than daily, looking for themes rather than reacting to individual entries. Does the child consistently struggle more on transition days versus mid-week? Do certain times of day prove more difficult? Are physical symptoms clustered around specific events? Do behaviors improve or worsen after a few days in each home? These patterns inform which strategies to try first and help parents understand their child's unique stress signature.

Importantly, tracking should have a defined purpose and endpoint. Parents are not creating permanent surveillance systems but rather gathering information for a specific period—perhaps four to six weeks—to understand their child's baseline responses to transitions. Once patterns become clear and parents implement responsive strategies, intensive tracking can ease, with parents returning to observation only if new concerns emerge or circumstances change significantly.

Learning to recognize dysregulation and anxiety in young children during custody transitions is not about achieving perfect observation or catching every signal before distress appears.

It is about building awareness of what stress looks like in a specific child — understanding that the six-year-old who bounces off the walls on nights before custody exchanges is communicating something just as clearly as the three-year-old who clings and cries, or the eight-year-old who goes silent and compliant. These behaviors are not problems to eliminate but information to receive, signals from a stress response system working hard to manage more than it can comfortably hold.

The physical signs—sleep disruption, appetite changes, toileting regression, stomachaches—arrive before words because young children's bodies speak what their developing brains cannot yet articulate. The behavioral signals shift across developmental stages, with three-year-olds expressing distress through tantrums and clinginess, five-year-olds asking the same worried questions repeatedly, and seven-year-olds either exploding with rage or disappearing into quiet compliance.

Neither presentation is better or worse; both require the same attentive response from parents who understand that behavior is communication, not manipulation.

For neurologically different children, dysregulation appears through the lens of their unique neurological wiring. ADHD amplifies emotional volatility and planning and organizing abilities collapse during transitions. Autism shifts distress toward shutdown, rigidity, and intensified stimming rather than verbal expression.

Sensory processing differences transform ordinary environmental variations between homes into physically overwhelming experiences that drain regulatory capacity entirely. Recognizing these neurodivergent presentations prevents parents from misinterpreting neurological responses as defiance or willful difficulty, allowing them to offer regulation support rather than consequences for behaviors their child cannot control.

The quiet, compliant child deserves particular attention in any discussion of recognizing distress. These children—who pack their bags without complaint, who smile and say they are fine, who never create visible problems around transitions—may actually be carrying significant internalized anxiety that goes completely unnoticed until it reaches a breaking point. Their good behavior masks suffering rather than reflecting genuine ease.

Parents must look beyond surface compliance to notice subtle shifts in physical health, emotional engagement, sleep patterns, and the quality of their child's presence, understanding that silence does not equal okayness.

Tracking patterns without panic provides the structure parents need to distinguish isolated difficult moments from genuine patterns requiring intervention. Simple observation tools—brief transition logs capturing basic information about behaviors and physical symptoms around custody exchanges—build clarity without creating surveillance systems that add to parental overwhelm.

The goal is noticing themes over time: Does the child consistently struggle more on transition days? Do certain physical symptoms cluster around specific events? Do behaviors improve after a few days in each home? These patterns inform responsive strategies while reducing the cognitive load of trying to remember details across weeks of emotionally intense parenting.

Recognition is the foundation, not the destination. Seeing that a child is dysregulated does not mean parents have failed or that the divorce is causing irreparable harm.

It means the child is having a normal response to significant life stress and needs support returning to regulation—support that becomes possible only when parents first notice the distress beneath the behavior.

The chapters that follow build on this foundation, offering concrete trauma-informed strategies for the before, during, and after phases of transitions, specialized support for neurodivergent children, and approaches for creating consistency even when co-parent cooperation remains impossible. But all of those strategies begin here, with parents who have learned to see what their child's body and behavior are trying to tell them.

# CHAPTER 3

# <u>Before, During, and After</u>
## Trauma-Informed Co-Parenting Strategies for Peaceful Transitions Between Households

The hardest part of shared parenting isn't always the big decisions about schools or schedules—it's often the ten minutes before your child walks out the door. It's the moment when your five-year-old's face crumples as she zips her backpack, or when your seven-year-old suddenly can't find his shoes, even though they've been sitting by the door all morning.

These moments—the actual transitions between your home and your co-parent's—are where theory meets reality, where all your intentions about staying calm and putting your child first get tested by your own racing heart and your child's big feelings. They're also the moments when your child is watching most carefully, reading your face and your body language to figure out if this change is safe, if both homes are okay, if they're allowed to love both parents without betraying anyone.

To help you navigate these critical moments with more confidence and clarity, this chapter breaks down the transition process into three manageable phases: before, during, and after. Each phase has its own emotional landscape, its own challenges, and its own opportunities to help your child feel secure. Understanding these phases helps you move from reacting in the moment to responding with intention, even when you're exhausted, even when your co-parent just sent a text that made your stomach drop, even when your child is melting down in the driveway.

The strategies in this chapter are designed to work within your own household and your own interactions with your child. They don't require your co-parent to cooperate, agree, or even understand what you're doing. They focus on what you can control: your own preparation, your own words, your own nervous system, and the environment you create in your home.

This matters because many parents reading this are navigating high-conflict situations where coordination feels impossible, where every interaction with an ex-partner is fraught, where the other household operates by completely different rules or values.

You'll learn specific language to use before your child leaves—words that prepare without creating anxiety, that acknowledge feelings without amplifying them. You'll discover what actually helps during the handoff moment itself, including how to stay calm when you're face-to-face with someone who may be trying to provoke you, and how to read your child's signals in real time. And you'll gain tools for the settling-in period after your child arrives at your home, when their nervous system needs support to shift gears and feel safe in this space again.

Throughout this chapter, you'll find adaptations for neurodivergent children who experience transitions with heightened intensity.

Children with ADHD often struggle with the planning and organization skills demands of packing and preparing, becoming overwhelmed by decisions and transitions between activities. Autistic children may need more concrete information about what's happening and when, along with sensory supports that help them manage the physical experience of moving between spaces. Highly sensitive children pick up on parental stress with particular acuity and may need extra reassurance that the adults are okay even when feelings are big.

The goal isn't perfection—and that's important to remember from the start. You will have handoffs that don't go smoothly. You will say things you wish you'd said differently. Your child will have hard days that no amount of preparation prevents.

What matters is building a foundation of predictability and emotional safety over time, so that even when individual transitions are difficult, your child knows what to expect from you and trusts that you can handle their feelings without falling apart.

This chapter gives you a roadmap for those everyday moments that feel so hard—not because they should be easy, but because you deserve to know what actually helps when you're standing in the doorway watching your child's face as they prepare to leave.

# The Before Phase: Preparing Your Child (and Yourself) for the Transition Without Creating Anxiety

The preparation phase begins well before your child's backpack appears by the door. It starts with your own stress response system—the tightness in your chest when you check the calendar and see tomorrow is a transition day, the way your shoulders creep toward your ears when you think about the exchange.

Children ages three through eight are extraordinarily attuned to parental stress, reading faces and body language long before they understand words. When a parent approaches a transition already flooded with anxiety, children absorb that signal as evidence that something dangerous is about to happen.

Preparing yourself means acknowledging what you're actually feeling—grief, anger, resentment toward your ex-partner, worry about what happens in the other home—and then creating enough space between those feelings and your child's experience that you can show up steady.

This doesn't require pretending everything is fine or achieving perfect calm. It means recognizing when your own distress is rising and using simple regulation techniques before your child enters the room. Take three slow breaths while standing at the kitchen sink, then spend a moment physically grounding yourself by feeling your feet on the floor. Remind yourself that your child needs you calm more than they need you to control what happens next.

For children, preparation works best when it's concrete, predictable, and emotionally neutral. Young children don't benefit from lengthy explanations or advance warnings that stretch across days, which can actually increase anxiety by creating prolonged anticipation. Instead, effective preparation happens in the twenty-four hours before a transition, using simple language that matches the child's developmental stage.

For three- and four-year-olds, preparation might sound like this at breakfast on transition day: "After your nap today, you'll go to Daddy's house. You'll sleep there tonight and tomorrow night, and then you'll come back here." Pair these words with a visual—pointing to a calendar with pictures, showing two fingers for two nights—because preschoolers understand concrete representations better than abstract time concepts. The tone matters as much as the words—use the same calm, matter-of-fact voice you'd use to describe what's for lunch.

Five- and six-year-olds can handle slightly more information and often want to know what comes next in both locations. "Tomorrow after school, I'll pick you up and we'll go to Mom's house. You'll have dinner there, do your bedtime routine, and sleep in your room at her place. On Saturday morning, you'll have breakfast with Mom." This age group benefits from knowing the immediate sequence without overwhelming detail about the entire week ahead.

Seven- and eight-year-olds may ask direct questions or express worries, and preparation includes space for those feelings without amplifying them. When a child says, "I don't want to go," the response isn't dismissal or over-reassurance, but acknowledgment: "I hear you. Sometimes transitions feel hard. And you're going to be okay. Both homes are safe places for you." This validates the feeling while providing the steady message that you can hold your child's distress without falling apart.

Neurodivergent children often need adapted preparation approaches. Children with ADHD benefit from breaking preparation into small, manageable steps rather than one overwhelming instruction—"First, get your backpack. Now, put in your stuffed animal"—with physical proximity and gentle redirection when attention wanders.

Autistic children may need more detailed information about exactly what will happen and when, along with visual schedules that reduce uncertainty.

Highly sensitive children pick up on unspoken tension and may need explicit reassurance: "I'm feeling some big feelings today, and that's okay. You're safe, and this transition will go just fine."

The preparation phase isn't about eliminating all difficulty. It's about creating enough predictability and emotional steadiness that your child approaches the transition knowing what to expect and trusting that you can handle whatever feelings arise.

## The During Phase: Managing the Handoff Moment with Calm and Consistency, Even in High-Conflict Situations

The handoff itself—the actual moment when your child moves from your care to your co-parent's—is where all your preparation either holds or unravels.

This is the moment your child is watching most intently, reading both adults' faces and bodies to determine whether this transition is safe or threatening. Young children regulate their own nervous systems by co-regulating with their caregivers, which means your child's ability to stay calm during the exchange depends significantly on your ability to remain grounded, even when facing a co-parent who may be hostile, unpredictable, or deliberately provocative.

The first principle of managing the handoff is brevity. Exchanges should be kept to two minutes or less, focused entirely on the child rather than adult logistics or grievances. Long conversations at the door create opportunities for conflict to surface in front of the child and signal to the child that something complicated and potentially unsafe is happening between the adults.

When a parent needs to communicate information—medication instructions, a change in the next pickup time—this should happen via text or email before the handoff, using brief, factual language that avoids emotional content or blame.

During the actual exchange, the parent's physical presence and tone communicate more than words. Stand with relaxed shoulders. Maintain a neutral facial expression and use a calm voice, even when internally distressed. These actions provide the child with visual and auditory signals that this moment is manageable.

When a co-parent arrives and tension is palpable, the calm parent can focus their attention on the child rather than engaging with the other adult. Simple phrases directed to the child work well: "Here's your backpack. I'll see you on Wednesday. I love you." Keep these words concrete, predictable, and emotionally steady—neither overly effusive nor anxious.

High-conflict situations require additional boundaries to protect children from witnessing adult hostility. When a co-parent attempts to engage in conflict—making a critical comment, questioning a parenting decision, or expressing anger—the most helpful response is often no response. Disengaging doesn't mean ignoring the child; it means refusing to participate in adult conflict while the child is present. You might acknowledge the co-parent with a brief nod, then turn your full attention back to your child, showing them that their emotional experience is what matters most.

For neurodivergent children, the handoff moment may require specific accommodations.

Children with ADHD often struggle with the abrupt shift in attention and environment, benefiting from a brief physical grounding activity before leaving—putting on shoes together, carrying a specific item to the car, or a quick hand squeeze that provides sensory input and connection.

Autistic children may need the handoff to follow an exact sequence every time: parent walks child to the door, child picks up backpack, parent says the same goodbye phrase, child walks to the other parent's car. Deviations from this sequence can trigger distress, so maintaining sameness even when the co-parent is unpredictable becomes essential.

Highly sensitive children often absorb tension between adults even when no words are spoken. For these children, a parent's internal regulation work before the handoff becomes critical. If a parent arrives at the exchange already flooded with anxiety or anger, the sensitive child will feel that energy and interpret it as danger. A brief pause before opening the door—three deep breaths, a moment of intentional grounding—can shift a parent's nervous system enough to show up steadier for the child.

When handoffs go poorly despite a parent's best efforts—when a child cries, when the co-parent creates a scene, when the moment feels chaotic—the parent's role is to remain the steady point. Children need to see that their parent can hold space for difficulty without collapsing, that big feelings don't break the adult, and that transitions can be hard and still be survivable. This consistency over time builds the child's trust that both homes are safe, even when the moment itself feels uncomfortable.

## The Settling-In Phase: Supporting Your Child's Nervous System as They Settle Into Your Home

The settling-in phase begins the moment your child walks through your door, and it's often more complex than parents anticipate. A child who seemed fine during the exchange may unravel twenty minutes later. A seven-year-old who appeared cheerful in the car might become defiant or withdrawn once inside. This isn't manipulation or misbehavior—it's emotional overwhelm surfacing in the one place the child feels safe enough to fall apart.

Young children's nervous systems operate on a principle called neuroception, a term coined by researcher Stephen Porges to describe how the body unconsciously assesses safety or threat. During transitions between homes, a child's nervous system has been working overtime to navigate change, manage big feelings, and read adult cues for danger.

When they arrive at your home, their system finally has permission to release the tension it's been holding, which often looks like challenging behavior rather than relief.

You don't need to master the neuroscience to help your child. Your calm presence already does more than theory ever could.

The first hour after arrival is critical for helping a child's nervous system calm down from the heightened state of transition. This doesn't mean forcing conversation about feelings or immediately launching into activities.

For many children, particularly those who are neurodivergent or highly sensitive, the most supportive approach is creating space for quiet, low-demand connection. This might look like sitting together on the couch without talking, offering a snack without requiring eye contact or conversation, or allowing the child to retreat to their room with a comfort item while the parent remains calmly nearby.

Physical regulation strategies help children's bodies shift from activation to safety. Deep pressure input—a firm hug if the child welcomes it, wrapping in a heavy blanket, or even pushing against a wall together—activates the parasympathetic nervous system, signaling to the body that it can begin to settle. Rhythmic, repetitive activities like coloring, playing with playdough, or bouncing on a yoga ball provide sensory input that supports regulation without requiring emotional processing the child may not yet be ready for.

For children with ADHD, the transition into your home may trigger hyperactivity or impulsivity as their nervous system struggles to shift gears. These children benefit from brief, structured physical activity immediately upon arrival—a few minutes of jumping jacks, a quick walk around the block, or throwing a ball back and forth—that burns off activation energy before expecting them to settle into quieter routines.

Autistic children often need predictable sensory environments and may require time in a designated calm space with familiar textures, sounds, or lighting that help their system recalibrate after the unpredictability of transition.

Avoid the common mistake of asking too many questions too soon. "How was it at Dad's?" or "Did you have fun?" can feel like interrogation to a child whose nervous system is already overwhelmed, and may create loyalty conflicts where the child worries that answering honestly will hurt one parent.

Instead, offer simple statements that communicate presence without demand: "I'm glad you're here. We're going to have dinner soon, and then we'll do your bedtime routine just like always."

Predictable routines in the settling-in phase provide the external structure that helps a child's internal system organize itself. When a child knows that arrival always includes the same sequence—shoes off, backpack in the same spot, hand washing, snack at the kitchen table—their nervous system can relax into the familiarity rather than scanning for what might be different or unsafe. This consistency matters more than the specific activities; what helps is the sameness, the reliability, the message that this home operates in ways the child can predict and trust.

Some children will need to reconnect through play rather than words, using toys or drawing to process what they're feeling without direct conversation. Others will chatter nonstop, filling the space with noise as a way to manage internal anxiety. Both responses are normal, and both require the parent's calm presence more than any specific intervention—the steady message that whatever the child brings home, the parent can hold it without falling apart.

# Trauma-Informed Communication: What to Say (and Not Say) Before, During, and After Transitions

The words parents use during transitions carry more weight than most realize. Young children ages three through eight are building their understanding of what divorce means, what two homes means, and whether they're safe in this new reality largely through the language their parents choose in these vulnerable moments. Children in this age range are concrete thinkers who interpret language literally and absorb emotional tone even more than content—meaning that what you say, and how you say it, directly shapes your child's sense of security during transitions.

Trauma-informed communication prioritizes the child's emotional safety above all else. It acknowledges that transitions between homes can activate stress responses in young children, and that the language surrounding these moments either supports regulation or amplifies emotional overwhelm. This approach focuses on creating predictability, validating feelings without intensifying them, and maintaining emotional steadiness even when the parent feels anything but steady inside.

### What to Say Before Transitions

Effective preparation language is concrete, calm, and developmentally appropriate. For three- and four-year-olds, this sounds like: "After lunch, you'll go to Daddy's house. You'll sleep there two times, then come back here." Pairing words with visual cues—holding up two fingers, pointing to pictures on a calendar—helps preschoolers grasp abstract time concepts. The tone should match the energy used to describe any other part of the day: matter-of-fact, warm, and unworried.

Five- and six-year-olds benefit from slightly more sequence information: "Tomorrow after school, Dad will pick you up. You'll have dinner at his house, do your bedtime routine there, and sleep in your room at Dad's. I'll see you Saturday morning." This age group wants to know what comes next without being overwhelmed by details stretching too far into the future.

Seven- and eight-year-olds may express resistance or worry directly, and preparation includes space for those feelings: "I hear that you don't want to go. Transitions can feel hard. And you're going to be okay. Both homes are safe places for you." This language validates the emotion while providing the steady message that the parent trusts the child's ability to manage the transition.

What not to say: Avoid language that expresses your own distress about the separation—"I'm going to miss you so much" or "I hate when you have to leave"—which can signal to your child that the transition is dangerous or wrong. Avoid asking the child to reassure you—"You'll be good for Daddy, right?" or "You still love me best, don't you?"—which places emotional labor on the child that doesn't belong to them.

## What to Say During Transitions

The exchange moment requires brevity and calm. Effective goodbye language is warm but confident: "I love you. Have a good time. I'll see you Wednesday." This communicates affection without clinging, and certainty without anxiety. If a child resists, acknowledge the feeling without collapsing: "I see you're upset. That's okay. You're safe with Dad, and I'll be here when you come back."

What not to say: Avoid prolonged, emotional goodbyes that signal danger—"I don't know how I'll survive without you" or tearful clinging. Avoid criticizing the other parent or making the child responsible for adult feelings—"Be brave for me" or "Don't let your mother upset you."

## What to Say After Transitions

When the child returns, greet them warmly without interrogation: "I'm glad you're home. I missed you." Allow space for the child to share if they want to, without pressure: "If you want to tell me about your time with Mom, I'd love to hear. And if you just want to play quietly for a bit, that's okay too." If the child shares something difficult, listen without judgment: "That sounds hard. Tell me more about how you felt."

What not to say: Avoid pumping for information—"What did you do at Dad's? Did he ask about me?"—or criticizing based on what the child reports—"Your mom let you stay up that late? That's ridiculous." These responses teach children that sharing their experience creates conflict, and they'll stop trusting parents with the truth of their lives between homes.

# Adapting the Three-Phase Framework for Neurodivergent Children: Executive Function Support, Sensory Regulation, and Extended Processing Time

Neurodivergent children experience the three-phase transition framework with intensified challenges that require specific adaptations to support their unique neurological processing. Children with ADHD, autism, sensory processing differences, and high sensitivity navigate transitions between homes with executive function demands, sensory overwhelm, and processing speeds that differ fundamentally from neurotypical peers. Understanding these differences allows parents to modify the before, during, and after phases in ways that honor how these children's brains and nervous systems actually work, rather than expecting them to adapt to approaches designed for neurotypical development.

## Executive Function Support in the Preparation Phase

The before phase presents particular challenges for children with ADHD and other executive function differences. These children struggle with the cognitive demands of preparing for transitions—organizing belongings, sequencing tasks, managing time, and shifting attention from one activity to another. What looks like resistance or defiance is often genuine overwhelm when a child's brain cannot break down the abstract instruction "get ready to go to Dad's" into concrete, manageable steps.

Effective preparation for these children requires external scaffolding that replaces the internal executive function skills still developing. This means creating visual checklists with pictures for each step: put pajamas in backpack, add toothbrush, choose two toys, put backpack by door. The checklist stays in the same location every time, and the parent works through it alongside the child rather than expecting independent completion. For younger children ages three through five, this might mean physically handing them one item at a time. For seven- and eight-year-olds, it might mean sitting nearby while they work through the list, offering gentle redirection when attention wanders.

Time blindness—the difficulty perceiving how much time has passed or remains—means these children benefit from visual timers that show time as a shrinking colored disk rather than abstract numbers. Setting a timer for thirty minutes before departure and placing it where the child can see it provides concrete information their brain can process. Pairing the timer with a five-minute warning delivered calmly and physically close to the child helps bridge the gap between knowing a transition is coming and actually initiating the preparation sequence.

## Sensory Regulation During the Handoff

The during phase presents intense sensory challenges for children with autism, sensory processing disorders, and high sensitivity. The physical environment of a exchange—car doors closing, adult voices, the smell of a different vehicle, the visual stimulation of a parking lot or doorstep—can flood a child's nervous system with input they cannot filter or organize the way neurotypical children do.

These children need sensory supports built directly into the exchange moment. A transition bag that travels between homes might include noise-canceling headphones, a familiar textured object to hold, or a small, weighted lap pad that provides calming deep pressure input. Some children benefit from wearing the same "transition hoodie" every time, creating a sensory constant in an otherwise changing environment. Parents can coordinate with co-parents about these supports through brief, factual text messages—"She'll be wearing her headphones during pickup"—without requiring agreement about why these accommodations matter.

Autistic children particularly benefit from exact sameness in the exchange sequence. The exchange happens in the same location, the parent uses the same goodbye phrase every time, the child carries the same bag to the car. When co-parents cannot or will not maintain this consistency, the calm parent focuses on keeping their own side of the exchange identical each time, providing at least one predictable anchor point.

## Extended Processing Time in the Settling-in Phase

Neurodivergent children's nervous systems require significantly longer recovery periods after transitions than standard advice suggests. Where neurotypical children might settle within twenty to thirty minutes, children with ADHD, autism, or high sensitivity may need one to two hours of low-demand time before their system downregulates enough to engage in typical household activities or conversation.

This extended processing time isn't optional—it's neurological necessity. Parents create a designated decompression space where the child can engage in regulating sensory activities without social demands: listening to familiar music, using playdough, lying under a weighted blanket, or engaging in repetitive movement like swinging or rocking. The parent remains calmly available nearby without initiating conversation or asking questions about the other home, allowing the child's system to recalibrate at its own pace before reintegration into family routines begins.

Transitions between homes will never be perfectly smooth, and that's not the goal. The goal is creating enough predictability, emotional steadiness, and nervous system support that your child can navigate these moments without feeling unsafe—even when they feel hard. The three-phase framework in this chapter provides structure for what often feels chaotic: the preparation before your child leaves, the exchange moment itself, and the settling-in period after they arrive. Each phase has its own emotional landscape and its own opportunities to communicate safety to your child through your regulated presence, your consistent routines, and your willingness to hold their big feelings without falling apart.

What matters most across all three phases is what you can control within your own household and your own responses. You cannot dictate how your co-parent manages transitions, what they say to your child, or whether they understand the developmental and neurological needs driving your child's behavior.

You can control your own preparation—both the practical steps of helping your child pack and the internal work of managing your nervous system before the exchange. What you say and how you say it remains within your control: choose words that validate feelings without amplifying anxiety and provide reassurance without making promises you cannot keep.

You can also control the environment you create in your home during the after phase, building routines that help your child's body and brain shift from activation to safety at their own pace.

For neurodivergent children, these adaptations are not optional extras—they are essential infrastructure that allows these children to access the same sense of security that comes more easily to neurotypical peers. Planning and organization skills support during preparation, sensory accommodations during handoffs, and extended processing time after arrival honor how these children's brains actually work rather than expecting them to conform to neurotypical timelines and demands.

When parents implement these adaptations consistently within their own household, children begin to internalize the message that their needs are valid, that their nervous system responses make sense, and that at least one home understands how to help them regulate through difficulty.

The language you use during transitions teaches your child whether their feelings are acceptable, whether both homes are safe, and whether you can be trusted to tell them the truth without burdening them with adult conflict.

Trauma-informed communication prioritizes your child's emotional safety above your own distress, above your frustration with your co-parent, and above the urge to gather information about what happens in the other household.

When you greet your child after a transition with warmth rather than interrogation, when you acknowledge their resistance without collapsing into anxiety, and when you validate their experience without criticizing their other parent, you build trust that allows them to bring their whole selves home to you.

The work of supporting transitions is repetitive, unglamorous, and often invisible. It happens in the moment you pause to regulate yourself before opening the door for a handoff. It happens when you sit quietly next to your dysregulated seven-year-old instead of demanding they talk about their feelings. It happens when you maintain the same goodbye phrase every single time even though your child barely seems to notice. This consistency over time—not perfection in any single moment—creates the foundation of security that allows children to build genuine belonging across two homes.

You will have transitions that go poorly. Your child will have meltdowns you cannot prevent. You will say things you wish you could take back. What repairs the ruptures and builds resilience is your willingness to show up again the next time, to keep offering the steady presence your child needs, and to trust that your regulated, consistent responses matter more than any single difficult moment. The strategies in this chapter give you a roadmap for that showing up—not because transitions should be easy, but because you and your child deserve to know what actually helps when the moment feels hard.

CHAPTER 4

# Helping Neurodivergent Children Through Divorce
## Specialized Support for ADHD, Autism, and Sensitive Kids

Your eight-year-old with ADHD melts down for forty minutes every single time he has to pack his bag for his dad's house, unable to start the task, overwhelmed by the decisions, and flooded with emotions he can't name. Your six-year-old autistic daughter, who thrives on sameness, has started scripting the same phrases over and over on transition days, her body rigid with anxiety about the unpredictability of moving between homes.

These aren't just difficult transitions—these are children whose neurological differences make the already-hard work of moving between two homes exponentially more challenging, and the standard advice about "keeping things simple" or "staying positive" doesn't come close to addressing what they actually need.

If you're parenting a neurodivergent child through divorce or separation, you already know that what works for neurotypical children often falls short for yours. The visual schedule that helps most five-year-olds feel prepared might overwhelm your autistic son who needs to know not just *what* will happen but *exactly how long* each part will take and *precisely what* the car will smell like and *whether* the same cup will be at Dad's house.

The cheerful reminder that "it's almost time to go" might send your daughter with ADHD into a shame spiral because she still hasn't managed to find her shoes, brush her teeth, or remember what she was supposed to pack, and now she's behind again and everyone's waiting and she doesn't understand why her brain won't just *work*.

This chapter is written for parents who are navigating divorce with children whose brains are wired differently—children with ADHD, autism spectrum differences, dyslexia, sensory processing differences, or high sensitivity. These children experience transitions, change, emotional regulation, and the entire reality of living in two homes with an intensity that can be difficult for others to understand. Their needs are not more complicated because they're being difficult—their needs are different because their nervous systems, executive function, sensory processing, and emotional regulation work differently than neurotypical children's.

The challenge becomes even more complex when your co-parent doesn't understand, accommodate, or even believe in your child's neurodivergent needs. Perhaps your ex dismisses the ADHD diagnosis as an excuse for bad behavior, refuses to follow the sensory strategies that help your child with autism regulate, or insists that your highly sensitive son just needs to "toughen up" instead of receiving the gentle support his nervous system requires. You cannot control what happens in the other household, and that reality can feel devastating when you know your child needs specific supports to feel safe and regulated.

What you can control is what happens in your home—the routines you build, the language you use, the accommodations you provide, and the understanding you bring to your child's experience. This chapter will teach you how to adapt transition strategies specifically for children with neurological differences, how to support executive function challenges during packing and handoffs, how to create predictability for children who need sameness, how to address sensory regulation during the physical experience of moving between homes, and how to communicate about divorce and transitions when your child processes language, time, and emotions differently.

You'll learn concrete approaches that work within your own household regardless of whether your co-parent implements them, strategies that honor your child's neurological differences rather than trying to force them into neurotypical expectations, and ways to build the emotional safety and regulation support your child needs to navigate an inherently challenging situation. Your child's neurodivergence doesn't make them broken or unable to adjust—it means they need you to understand how their brain works and meet them where they are with the specific supports that actually help.

# Understanding the Neurodivergent Experience of Divorce: How ADHD, Autism, and Sensory Differences Amplify Transition Stress

To understand why neurodivergent children struggle so intensely with divorce transitions, parents need to recognize how neurological differences fundamentally change the experience of moving between homes. What feels manageable to a neurotypical child—packing a bag, saying goodbye, adjusting to a different bedtime routine—can overwhelm a neurodivergent child's nervous system in ways that aren't about willfulness or poor adjustment. These children aren't being more difficult; their brains process an inherently difficult situation through different neurological pathways.

Research consistently shows that children with ADHD, autism spectrum differences, and sensory processing challenges face elevated stress during family transitions compared to their neurotypical peers. Studies indicate that families with neurodivergent children experience higher divorce rates, with parents of children diagnosed with ADHD showing divorce rates approximately 75% higher within ten years of the child's birth compared to families with neurotypical children, and families with autistic children facing similarly elevated separation likelihood. This isn't because these children cause divorce, but because the intensive support needs and lack of adequate resources can create additional strain on parental relationships—and when those relationships end, the children face transition challenges with fewer internal resources to manage them.

Statistics describe patterns, not destinies. Your child's outcome is shaped most by the steadiness and support you provide now.

If this section feels intense, that's understandable. You don't need to absorb it all at once. Your presence and consistency matter far more than any statistic.

## Executive Function and the Invisible Overwhelm

Children with ADHD struggle with executive function—the brain's ability to plan, organize, initiate tasks, and shift between activities. For these children, the instruction to "pack your bag for Dad's house" isn't a simple task; it's a complex multi-step process their brain cannot break down without support. They must remember what items to pack, locate those items in different rooms, make decisions about what's needed, organize items into the bag, and do all of this while managing the emotional weight of leaving one parent.

Executive function challenges mean they become stuck before starting, forget steps midway through, or melt down from the cognitive load—not because they don't want to go, but because their brain cannot sequence the task while simultaneously processing the emotional transition.

Time perception differences compound this struggle. Children with ADHD experience time inconsistently; "we're leaving in ten minutes" may feel like an immediate demand or like an eternity, making it nearly impossible to prepare emotionally or practically. The transition happens to them rather than with them, creating a perpetual sense of being rushed, behind, or caught off-guard.

Take a breath here. None of this means your child is incapable of adjusting— it means their brain needs clearer structure and support during change.

## Autism and the Disruption of Predictability

Autistic children depend on sameness and predictability to regulate their nervous systems in a world that often feels overwhelming and unpredictable. Divorce shatters this foundation. Even when parents create visual schedules and maintain routines, the fundamental reality remains: the child's world has changed in ways they didn't choose and cannot control. Two homes mean two sets of sensory environments, two different ways of doing bedtime, two variations of what "dinner" means—and for a child whose brain seeks patterns and consistency to feel safe, this variability creates constant low-level stress.

Autistic children may also struggle with perspective-taking and understanding the abstract concept that both parents still love them even when living separately. The concrete reality—Mom is here, Dad is not—can override verbal reassurances. Transitions require them to shift not just locations but entire mental frameworks about where they belong and who is available, a cognitive demand that intensifies anxiety.

## Sensory Processing and Physical Overwhelm

Children with sensory processing differences experience transitions as physical assaults on their nervous system. The car ride smells different, the other house sounds different, and the sheets feel different. The soap, the lighting, the ambient noise level—every environmental shift registers as significant sensory input requiring processing and adjustment. What neurotypical children might not consciously notice, sensory-sensitive children experience as a constant barrage of stimulation that depletes their regulation capacity before they even walk through the door.

These children aren't overreacting to small differences—their nervous systems genuinely process sensory information with greater intensity, making environmental changes feel destabilizing rather than merely different.

## Executive Function Support for ADHD Children: Breaking Down Packing, Transitions, and Two-Home Routines Into Manageable Steps

For children with ADHD, the instruction to "pack your bag for Dad's house" isn't a single task—it's a cascade of executive function demands their brain struggles to sequence without external support. These children face deficits in organization, planning, time management, task initiation, and cognitive flexibility that make transitions between homes exponentially more challenging than for neurotypical peers.

Research consistently demonstrates that children with ADHD experience significant executive function impairments that worsen under stress, and divorce ranks as one of the most stressful life events a child can experience.

The prefrontal cortex, which governs executive functioning, becomes overwhelmed when managing both the cognitive demands of transitions and the emotional weight of family change, leading to behavior regression, emotional dysregulation, and what can look like defiance but is actually neurological overwhelm.

Parents cannot simply tell an ADHD child to pack and expect follow-through—the brain's executive system requires scaffolding to break complex tasks into manageable steps. When the co-parent doesn't understand or accommodate these needs, dismissing struggles as laziness or poor parenting rather than recognizing the neurological reality, this support becomes even more critical. What parents can control is how they structure transitions within their own household, providing the external executive function support their child's brain cannot yet generate independently.

### Breaking Down Packing Into Visual, Sequential Steps

Packing overwhelms ADHD children because it requires holding multiple steps in working memory while making decisions, locating items, and managing the emotional reality of leaving. Parents can reduce this cognitive load by creating identical visual checklists for both homes—laminated cards with pictures showing each item needed (pajamas, toothbrush, favorite stuffed animal, school folder) that the child checks off with a dry-erase marker or stickers.

For children ages three through five, limit the list to five essential items with clear pictures. For ages six through eight, expand gradually to seven or eight items, grouped by category (clothes, toiletries, school items).

The checklist should live in the same location in each home—posted on the child's bedroom door or inside their backpack—so the routine becomes predictable. Parents work alongside the child initially, narrating each step: "First, we're finding pajamas. Where do pajamas live? Let's check that off. Next is your toothbrush." As the child develops competence, parents fade their involvement, moving from doing together to nearby supervision to independent completion with a final check-in.

Time perception differences mean ADHD children cannot accurately gauge how long packing takes or when they need to start. Parents should use visual timers showing time remaining in red, yellow, and green zones, beginning packing thirty minutes before departure rather than five. Breaking the task into timed segments—"We'll pack clothes for ten minutes, then take a movement break, then pack school things"—prevents the paralysis that comes from viewing packing as one overwhelming block.

## Simplifying Transitions With Predictable Rituals

Transitions trigger executive function lapses because they require cognitive flexibility—shifting from one set of expectations, routines, and environments to another. ADHD children benefit from identical pre-transition rituals that signal change is coming without requiring them to remember what happens next. This might include a specific goodbye routine: reviewing the visual schedule showing when they'll return, packing the transition comfort item that travels between homes, choosing a car snack from two options, and a consistent phrase like "See you on Wednesday after school."

Shared digital calendars with color-coded visuals help children see the pattern of transitions over time, building their understanding of the schedule's predictability. Parents should review the upcoming home's routine the night before: "Tomorrow after school, you'll go to Mom's. At Mom's, dinner happens at six, then bath, then two stories." This preview reduces the cognitive demand of remembering different household patterns while emotionally processing the transition.

## Establishing Manageable Two-Home Routines

Routines provide the external structure ADHD brains need to sustain executive skills like task persistence and organization. Parents should coordinate on core routine elements—morning wake-up sequences, homework time, bedtime—using similar visual supports in both homes even when the co-parent won't fully cooperate. A parent can create a picture schedule showing the morning routine (alarm, dress, breakfast, brush teeth, pack bag) and send a duplicate to the other household, knowing that even if it's not used there, the consistency in their own home builds the child's internal capacity for routine over time.

## Creating Predictability for Autistic Children: Visual Schedules, Transition Objects, and Honoring the Need for Sameness Across Two Homes

Autistic children depend on predictability and sameness to regulate their nervous systems in a world that often feels overwhelming and chaotic. When divorce disrupts the fundamental structure of their daily life, the loss of sameness can trigger profound anxiety that manifests as increased stimming, rigid adherence to remaining routines, meltdowns over seemingly minor changes, or withdrawal into scripted language and repetitive behaviors.

These aren't signs of poor adjustment—they're neurological responses to an environment that has become unpredictable in ways the child's brain finds genuinely threatening to their sense of safety.

Research consistently demonstrates that autistic children experience significantly elevated stress during family transitions, with routine disruption ranking among the most dysregulating experiences for children who rely on environmental consistency to manage sensory and emotional overwhelm. Courts and custody evaluators increasingly recognize that autistic children benefit from custody arrangements that prioritize stability, consistent schedules, and parental cooperation in maintaining similar routines across households. However, many parents face the reality that their co-parent doesn't understand or accommodate their child's need for sameness, dismissing it as rigidity that needs to be broken rather than a neurological requirement that deserves respect.

What parents can control is how they build predictability within their own household and what supports they provide to help their child navigate the unavoidable differences between two homes. Visual schedules, transition objects, and intentional efforts to replicate key routines become essential tools—not because they eliminate the difficulty of living in two places, but because they provide the external structure an autistic child's brain needs to process change without becoming completely overwhelmed.

## Visual Schedules That Make Time and Transitions Concrete

Autistic children often struggle with abstract concepts like time, making phrases like "you'll go to Dad's house on Friday" nearly meaningless without visual support.

A visual calendar using photographs—not just generic icons—of each parent's actual home, the child's bedroom in each location, and the parent's face creates concrete understanding of the custody pattern.

For children ages three through five, a simple weekly chart with two or three photos per day (morning location, parent, bedtime location) provides enough information without overwhelming. For ages six through eight, expand to include specific activities (school, therapy, dinner routine) that anchor each day's structure.

The calendar should be identical in both homes, posted at the child's eye level in a consistent location, and reviewed daily as part of a predictable routine—perhaps each morning at breakfast or each evening before bed. Parents should use the same language when referencing the schedule: "Let's check the calendar. Today is Tuesday. The calendar shows you're sleeping at my house tonight. Tomorrow is Wednesday, and you'll go to Mom's house after school." This repetition builds the child's ability to anticipate transitions rather than experiencing them as sudden disruptions.

Digital shared calendars work well when both parents cooperate, but when the co-parent won't participate, a parent can still create and maintain the visual schedule in their own home. The predictability the child experiences in one household builds their overall capacity to tolerate the unpredictability in the other, even when it's not ideal.

### Transition Objects That Carry Sameness Between Homes

Transition objects serve as physical anchors of continuity when the environment changes. These aren't just comfort items—they're sensory-consistent objects that signal safety across locations. A small photo album with pictures of both homes, both parents, the child's bedrooms, and important people travels in the child's backpack, available for review during car rides or moments of anxiety. A specific blanket, stuffed animal, or sensory toy that smells and feels the same provides regulatory support during the disorienting experience of moving between houses.

For autistic children, sameness means sensory sameness. Parents should coordinate on having identical items in both homes whenever possible — the same brand of toothpaste, the same color towels, the same bedtime books — recognizing that what seems like a minor detail to neurotypical perception registers as significant environmental change to an autistic child's sensory system.

## Sensory Regulation Strategies: Supporting Highly Sensitive and Sensory-Processing Children Through the Physical Experience of Moving Between Households

When a sensory-sensitive child transitions between homes, they're not just moving locations—they're navigating a complete sensory environment shift that their nervous system registers as significant and often overwhelming.

The car smells different than it did last week. The sheets at Dad's house feel scratchy compared to the soft ones at Mom's. The refrigerator hums louder in one kitchen. The soap dispenser makes a different sound.

For children with sensory processing differences or high sensitivity, these aren't minor details they can ignore—they're physical experiences that demand neurological processing and can deplete regulation capacity before the child even unpacks their bag.

Research demonstrates that highly sensitive children and those with sensory processing challenges experience sensory input with greater intensity than their neurotypical peers, leading to faster overwhelm during environmental changes like household transitions.

These children aren't overreacting or being difficult—their nervous systems genuinely process sensory information differently, making what seems like a small environmental shift feel destabilizing rather than merely different.

When parents understand that sensory regulation isn't about toughening children up but about providing the specific supports their nervous system requires, they can create strategies that actually reduce transition distress.

Sensory overwhelm is not permanent harm. It is a nervous system working hard to adapt.

The challenge intensifies when co-parents maintain different sensory environments—one home is quiet and dimly lit while the other has overhead fluorescent lights and a television constantly playing, or one parent uses unscented laundry detergent while the other uses heavily fragranced products. Parents cannot always control what happens in the other household, but they can provide sensory supports within their own home and during the transition itself that help their child's nervous system manage the physical experience of moving between worlds.

## Creating Sensory Continuity Through Portable Regulation Tools

A transition kit that travels between homes provides sensory consistency when everything else changes. This isn't just a comfort item—it's a carefully selected collection of sensory tools that help the child regulate during the car ride and upon arrival. For younger children ages three through five, this might include a soft stuffed animal that smells familiar, a chewy necklace for oral sensory input, and noise-canceling headphones for car rides. For ages six through eight, expand to include fidget tools, a small photo album with pictures of both homes and both parents, and perhaps a playlist of calming music the child chooses.

The kit should contain items that address the child's specific sensory profile. For instance, children who seek deep pressure benefit from a small, weighted lap pad for car rides, while children sensitive to tactile input, a favorite soft blanket or toy that feels the same regardless of location is best. Children who regulate through movement might include a small squishy ball they can squeeze during the drive. Parents work with their child to identify what actually helps rather than guessing, asking questions like "What helps your body feel calm when things feel too loud?" or "What do you like to touch when you're feeling worried?"

## Providing Sensory Breaks Before, During, and After Transitions

Sensory-sensitive children need deliberate decompression time built into the transition process rather than rushing from one environment to another.

Before leaving for the other parent's home, parents can offer a sensory break—ten minutes of quiet time in a calm space, a warm bath, or gentle rocking—that allows the child's nervous system to prepare for change. During the car ride, parents minimize additional sensory input by keeping music low or off, avoiding busy routes when possible, and allowing the child to use their regulation tools without pressure to talk or engage.

Upon arrival at either home, children need downtime before expectations begin. A parent might say, "You just did the hard work of moving between houses. Your body needs some quiet time. You can play in your room, look at books, or snuggle on the couch for twenty minutes before dinner." This isn't avoidance—it's providing the sensory reset their nervous system requires to function in the new environment. For neurodivergent children, this decompression period may need to extend to thirty or forty minutes, and that's appropriate support rather than indulgence.

## Co-Regulation Through Calm Presence

Parents support sensory regulation not just through environmental modifications but through their own nervous system state. When a child becomes overwhelmed by sensory input during transitions, a parent's calm, grounded presence provides the external regulation the child's system needs. This might look like sitting quietly nearby without talking, offering gentle pressure through a hug if the child accepts touch, or simply breathing slowly and staying physically close. Parents cannot eliminate sensory challenges, but they can be the steady anchor that helps their child's nervous system return to baseline after sensory overwhelm.

Parenting a child with neurological differences through divorce requires a fundamental shift in how transitions are understood and supported. The strategies that work for neurotypical children—simple verbal reminders, basic visual schedules, cheerful reassurances—often fall short for children whose brains process executive function, sensory input, predictability, and emotional regulation through different neurological pathways. These children aren't struggling more because they're being difficult or because parents are doing something wrong. They're struggling more because the already-challenging work of moving between two homes places exponentially greater demands on nervous systems that are wired differently.

What this chapter has established is that children with neurological differences need specialized supports that honor how their specific brain works rather than expecting them to adapt to strategies designed for neurotypical development.

Children with ADHD need external executive function scaffolding—visual checklists, task breakdowns, time timers, and physical support during packing and transitions—because their prefrontal cortex cannot yet generate these organizational skills independently, especially under the stress of family change. Autistic children need concrete predictability through visual schedules with photographs, transition objects that carry sensory sameness between homes, and identical routines that reduce the cognitive load of navigating two different environments. Sensory-sensitive children need regulation tools that address their specific sensory profile, decompression time before and after transitions, and environmental modifications that prevent sensory overwhelm from depleting their capacity to cope.

The reality many parents face is that their co-parent doesn't understand, accommodate, or even believe in their child's neurodivergent needs. Perhaps the other household dismisses the ADHD diagnosis, refuses to implement sensory strategies, or insists that the autistic child just needs to be more flexible. This lack of cooperation doesn't mean parents are powerless. What happens in one home matters profoundly for a child's overall regulation and sense of safety, even when the other home provides inconsistent support. The visual schedule a parent maintains, the executive function scaffolding they provide, the sensory regulation tools they offer—these supports build the child's internal capacity over time, creating resilience that carries into all environments.

Parents should recognize that supporting a neurodivergent child through divorce is inherently more demanding than supporting a neurotypical child through the same transition. This isn't a reflection of parental inadequacy—it's acknowledgment of neurological reality. These children require more preparation time, more concrete information, more sensory accommodations, more emotional processing support, and more patience when regulation fails despite everyone's best efforts. The additional effort this requires is real, and parents deserve validation for the exhausting, often invisible work of translating a neurotypical world into supports their child's brain can actually use.

The communication adaptations discussed in this chapter—concrete language instead of abstract explanations, visual supports for time and emotions, extended processing time, and validation of literal interpretations—aren't just helpful additions to standard divorce conversations. They're essential modifications that determine whether a neurodivergent child can comprehend what's happening to their family and access the reassurance their parents are trying to provide. When parents meet their child where they are neurologically rather than where developmental norms suggest they should be, they create the foundation for genuine emotional safety rather than surface compliance that masks internal confusion and distress.

Your child's neurodivergence doesn't make them incapable of adjusting to two homes or destined for poor outcomes. It means they need you to understand how their brain works and provide the specific supports that actually help—supports you can implement in your own household regardless of what happens elsewhere, building the regulation skills and secure attachment that will carry them through this transition and beyond.

# CHAPTER 5

# <u>Two Homes, Two Worlds</u>
## Creating Consistency for Young Kids Without Co-Parent Cooperation in High-Conflict Situations

Your seven-year-old comes back from their other parent's house talking about staying up until ten o'clock and eating ice cream for breakfast, while you've spent months building a bedtime routine that finally helps them sleep. Your five-year-old asks why they have to brush their teeth at your house when they don't have to at the other parent's house, their voice already carrying the weight of confusion about which rules are real.

These moments disrupt the careful structure you've been trying to build. You've read the advice about co-parenting consistency, about presenting a united front, about keeping rules the same across both households. And then you face the reality: your co-parent doesn't answer your texts about bedtime, serves dinner at nine o'clock, or tells your child that your rules are "too strict." You cannot control what happens in the other home. You cannot make your ex-partner follow the same routines, use the same language, or prioritize the same values. And the powerlessness of that reality can feel overwhelming when you're trying so hard to give your child stability.

This chapter acknowledges what many co-parenting books gloss over: sometimes you are doing this alone. Sometimes the other parent undermines, dismisses, or simply operates from a completely different playbook. Sometimes the differences between homes aren't just about minor variations in snack choices—they're fundamental differences in structure, safety, or emotional attunement. And sometimes those differences feel concerning to your child's well-being in ways that keep you awake at night.

But here is what this chapter will help you understand: you cannot create perfect consistency across two homes, and your child does not need perfect consistency to feel safe and develop healthy regulation. What your child needs is one home where things are predictable, where emotions are held steadily, where they can exhale and know what comes next. They need one parent who stays calm when they're confused, who doesn't ask them to carry messages or make judgments, who helps them hold two different realities without feeling torn apart by them. That parent can be you, in your home, regardless of what happens anywhere else.

Young children ages three through eight are building their internal sense of how the world works—what they can count on, who will catch them when they fall, how to manage big feelings in their small bodies. They are not looking for perfection. They are looking for patterns they can predict, adults who stay steady when things feel chaotic, and reassurance that they are loved in both places even when those places feel like different planets. You can provide that foundation within your own four walls, and it will matter more than you might believe possible right now.

This chapter will teach you how to build that single-home foundation—how to create routines, rules, and emotional constants that work independently of what your co-parent does or doesn't do. You'll learn specific language for talking to your child about differences between homes without criticizing the other parent or asking your child to choose sides. You'll discover how to support your child's regulation when they return from a chaotic or unpredictable environment, and how to let go of what you cannot control without letting go of your child's emotional safety.

For parents of neurodivergent children—those with ADHD, autism, dyslexia, or high sensitivity—this chapter offers additional strategies for children who struggle intensely with inconsistency and need extra scaffolding to navigate two different sets of expectations. These children often need more explicit support to manage the cognitive load of switching between different rules, routines, and sensory environments.

You cannot control the other home. But you can build something sturdy, warm, and reliable in yours. And that will be enough.

# What Consistency Really Means for Young Children: Building Internal Safety When External Circumstances Are Unpredictable

When parents hear the word "consistency," they often picture two households operating in perfect synchronization—same bedtimes, same rules about screen time, same consequences for misbehavior, same language about feelings. This vision of consistency feels impossible when co-parenting is difficult, and the gap between the ideal and reality can leave parents feeling defeated before they begin. But this understanding of consistency misses what young children actually need to feel safe.

For children ages three through eight, consistency is not about identical external circumstances across two homes. It is about building an internal sense of safety—a felt experience in the body and nervous system that says, "I know what happens next here. I can predict how the adults will respond. I am safe enough to relax." This internal safety develops when a child experiences reliable patterns within at least one environment, even when patterns differ between environments.

Neuroscience research on early childhood stress and regulation confirms that predictable routines activate the parasympathetic nervous system, which helps children's bodies move out of fight-or-flight responses and into states where learning, connection, and emotional processing become possible.

When a four-year-old knows that bedtime in your home always includes the same sequence—pajamas, teeth, two stories, lights out—their nervous system begins to anticipate and prepare for sleep before the routine even starts. This neurological predictability matters more than whether bedtime happens at the same time or in the same way at her other parent's house.

Young children in this age range are developing their understanding of cause and effect, learning to predict outcomes based on patterns they observe. When those patterns hold steady in at least one environment, children can begin to develop what developmental psychologists call an internal locus of control—a sense that the world has order, that their behavior connects to predictable responses, and that they have some agency in managing their own experience. This internal framework travels with them between homes, even when the external circumstances shift dramatically.

The elements that build this internal safety are specific and manageable within a single household. A consistent morning routine—wake up, breakfast, getting dressed in the same order—creates a predictable start regardless of which home the child woke up in.

Consistent emotional responses from a parent—calm acknowledgment of big feelings, the same phrases of reassurance, predictable repair after conflict—teach a child that this adult can be counted on to stay steady. Consistent rules within your home—we use gentle hands, we clean up before screen time, we talk about feelings instead of throwing things—create boundaries that help children feel contained and safe, even if those rules don't exist elsewhere.

For neurodivergent children, this within-home consistency becomes even more critical. Children with ADHD benefit enormously from routines that reduce the executive function load of decision-making—when the morning sequence never changes, they don't have to hold multiple steps in working memory or make choices while already dysregulated.

Autistic children, who often experience intense distress when expectations shift unpredictably, find regulation through sameness within one environment, even when they cannot control what happens in the other.

Highly sensitive children, whose nervous systems register every environmental change, need the predictability of one home's rhythms to recover from the sensory and emotional intensity of transitions.

Building consistency within your own home does not require your co-parent's participation, permission, or agreement. What it does require is your commitment to creating reliable patterns that your child's nervous system can learn to trust. Over time, this singular foundation of safety becomes something your child carries internally—a felt sense that at least one part of their world is steady, predictable, and safe enough to exhale into.

## The Single-Home Foundation: Creating Predictable Routines, Rules, and Emotional Anchors Within Your Household That Work Independently

Building a single-home foundation begins with understanding that predictability within a single household creates neurological safety for young children, even when the other household operates entirely differently.

This foundation rests on three interconnected elements: routines that reduce cognitive load, rules that provide containment, and emotional anchors that communicate unconditional presence. Each element functions independently of what happens elsewhere, giving parents concrete control over their child's experience within their own four walls.

Predictable routines work by allowing a child's nervous system to anticipate what comes next, reducing the constant vigilance that characterizes stress responses. For children ages three through eight, routines should cover the major transition points of the day—waking up, mealtimes, after-school or after-daycare time, bedtime—because these moments naturally carry higher emotional intensity. A morning routine might always follow the same sequence: wake up, use the bathroom, get dressed, eat breakfast, brush teeth. The specific activities matter less than the consistency of the order. When a six-year-old experiences the same breakfast-then-dressing sequence every morning in your home, their brain learns to relax into this pattern, even if the other home follows a different order.

For neurodivergent children, routines require additional scaffolding.

Children with ADHD benefit from picture schedules posted at eye level that break each routine into individual steps with pictures or icons, reducing the short-term memory demand of remembering what comes next.

Autistic children often need advance notice before routine changes and may require the same routine to happen in the exact same physical location each time—always brushing teeth at the same sink, always putting shoes on while sitting in the same spot.

Highly sensitive children may need routines that include sensory regulation breaks, such as five minutes of quiet time with a weighted lap pad after the stimulation of getting home from school.

Rules within one household provide the boundaries that help children feel contained and safe. These rules do not need to match the other home's rules to be effective. A parent might establish clear expectations: we use kind words when we're frustrated, we put toys away before screen time, we sit at the table during meals.

The key is consistent enforcement within this home, paired with calm, predictable responses when rules are broken. A four-year-old who throws a toy in anger needs to know that the response will be the same every time — perhaps a calm statement like "Throwing can hurt someone. Let's take a break together," followed by the same brief time-in process. This predictability teaches the child that this adult can be trusted to stay steady, which builds internal regulation over time.

When rules differ between homes, young children need simple, non-judgmental language that acknowledges the difference without asking them to take sides. A parent might say, "At this house, we always brush teeth before bed. I know it might be different at Dad's house, and that's okay. Different houses can have different rules. At this house, this is how we do it." This language validates the child's reality without criticism, helping them hold two different sets of expectations without feeling torn.

Emotional anchors are the relational consistencies that communicate to a child: you are safe with me, I will stay calm when you cannot, your feelings are welcome here. These anchors show up in repeated phrases—"I'm right here," "You're safe," "We'll figure this out together"—and in consistent emotional responses. When a seven-year-old returns from the other home dysregulated and snaps at their parent, an emotional anchor might sound like, "I can see you're having a hard time. I'm not going anywhere. When you're ready, I'm here." The steadiness of this response, repeated across many difficult moments, becomes something the child internalizes: this parent will not collapse, retaliate, or disappear when things are hard.

For neurodivergent children, emotional anchors may need to be more concrete and less reliant on verbal processing. A child with autism might benefit from a physical anchor—a specific blanket that lives in the same spot, always available for regulation. A child with ADHD might need movement-based anchoring, such as a parent who always offers a walk around the block when big feelings hit. These adaptations honor how different nervous systems find safety.

## Talking to Young Children About Differences Between Homes: Scripts and Approaches That Validate Reality Without Criticism or Loyalty Conflicts

When your child asks why bedtime differs between houses or why screen time rules don't match, they're not seeking a detailed explanation of parenting philosophies or disagreement history. They are asking a simpler, deeper question: Is it okay that these two places I love are not the same? Can I belong in both without having to choose? The way a parent responds to these questions shapes whether a child learns to hold complexity with ease or carries the weight of divided loyalty.

The goal of talking about differences between homes is not to explain them away, justify your approach, or subtly communicate that the other home is lacking. The goal is to validate your son or daughter's reality—to acknowledge that yes, things are different, and that difference does not require them to judge, choose, or carry messages between parents. Research on children's adjustment to divorce consistently shows that loyalty conflicts—the felt pressure to align with one parent against the other—are among the most damaging aspects of family separation for young children. When parents criticize each other or ask children to compare homes, children experience this as an impossible choice between two people they need and love.

Effective scripts for talking about differences share several key elements. They name the difference neutrally, without judgment or emotional charge. They normalize the existence of two different ways of doing things. They reassure the child that both homes care about their well-being. And they close the loop—they do not leave the conversation open-ended in a way that invites the child to problem-solve, take sides, or carry the topic back to the other parent.

A parent might say: "At Dad's house, bedtime is at eight-thirty. At this house, bedtime is at seven-thirty. Different homes have different routines, and that's okay. Both routines help you get the sleep you need." This language is factual, brief, and complete. It does not invite comparison—"Which do you like better?"—or criticism—"I think earlier is healthier." It simply states what is true and offers reassurance that the child does not need to reconcile the difference.

When a five-year-old says, "Mommy lets me have iPad time before bed," a parent might respond: "That's how Mommy does it at her house. At this house, we do quiet books before bed. You get to do it both ways." The phrase "you get to do it both ways" reframes difference as abundance rather than conflict. The child is not being asked to decide which way is right. They are being told that both ways exist, both are acceptable, and they can participate in both without betraying anyone.

For neurodivergent children who process language literally or struggle with ambiguity, these scripts may need additional clarity. An autistic child might need explicit reassurance: "The rule at this house is we brush teeth after breakfast. The rule at Dad's house might be different. Both rules are real. You follow this rule here, and Dad's rule there. That is how two-home families work." The concrete structure—this rule here, that rule there—provides cognitive scaffolding that reduces anxiety about inconsistency.

Children with ADHD, who may struggle with rule-switching due to executive function challenges, benefit from visual reminders. A parent might create a simple chart: "Rules at This House" with pictures posted where the child can see it. When the child references the other home's rules, the parent can say, "That's Dad's house rules. Here are our house rules," and point to the chart. This externalizes the rule structure, reducing the cognitive load of holding two sets of expectations in working memory.

When differences feel significant—one home has structure, the other does not; one home is safe, the other is chaotic—parents face the challenge of validating their child's experience without badmouthing the co-parent. A parent might say: "I notice you seem really tired when you come back from Dad's. It's hard when bedtimes are different. At this house, we'll make sure you get rest." This acknowledges the child's reality, offers comfort, and focuses on what the parent can control without criticizing what they cannot.

## Supporting Neurodivergent Children Who Need Sameness: Extra Scaffolding for ADHD, Autistic, and Highly Sensitive Children Navigating Inconsistent Expectations

Neurodivergent children—those with ADHD, autism, or high sensitivity—experience inconsistency between homes with an intensity that neurotypical children do not.

For these children, differences in routines, sensory environments, and expectations are not minor inconveniences to adjust to; they are neurological disruptions that can trigger dysregulation, anxiety, and a profound sense of unsafety.

When a seven-year-old autistic child knows that bedtime at one home follows a precise sequence—bath, pajamas, three specific books, lights out at exactly eight o'clock—and the other household has no bedtime routine at all, their nervous system does not simply "adjust." It remains in a state of hypervigilance, unable to predict what comes next, unable to relax into the patterns that allow her brain to feel safe.

Children with ADHD struggle with inconsistent expectations because their executive function systems—the brain networks responsible for planning, organizing, and shifting between tasks—are already working harder than their neurotypical peers.

When rules change between homes, these children must hold two entirely different sets of behavioral expectations in short-term memory, switch between them during transitions, and inhibit the impulse to follow the "wrong" rule in the "wrong" house.

This cognitive load is exhausting and often impossible, leading to what parents perceive as defiance or carelessness but is actually neurological overwhelm.

Highly sensitive children, whose nervous systems process sensory and emotional information more deeply, experience the differences between homes as a constant recalibration. The lighting, the noise level, the emotional temperature of each household, the way adults respond to distress—all of these differences require the child's nervous system to continuously adapt rather than settle. For these children, inconsistency is not just confusing; it is physiologically depleting.

When co-parents cannot or will not create consistency together, parents must provide extra scaffolding within their own home that helps neurodivergent children manage the reality of two different worlds. This scaffolding is not about making the child tougher or more flexible. It is about building external supports that compensate for the neurological challenges these children face when their environment lacks the sameness their brains require to function well.

Visual supports become essential tools. A visual schedule that shows the routine in this home—using pictures, icons, or simple words—externalizes the structure so the child does not have to hold it all in memory. For an autistic child, this schedule might need to be identical every single day, posted in the same location, reviewed at the same time each morning. For a child with ADHD, the schedule might include checkboxes the child can physically mark off, providing the dopamine reward of task completion that helps sustain attention and motivation through multi-step routines.

Transition objects—items that travel between homes and belong only to the child—provide sensory and emotional anchoring. A specific blanket, a small stuffed animal, a favorite book that lives in the child's backpack can serve as a portable piece of sameness when everything else shifts. For highly sensitive children, these objects often carry sensory comfort—a particular texture, smell, or weight that helps regulate their nervous system during the disorientation of moving between homes.

Explicit verbal scaffolding helps neurodivergent children navigate rule differences without internalizing the inconsistency as chaos. A parent might say, "At this house, we always sit at the table for meals. I know it's different at Dad's house. When you're here, this is the rule. Your brain might feel confused about which rule to follow, and that's okay. I'll remind you gently." This language names the cognitive challenge, normalizes the confusion, and reassures the child that the adult will provide external support rather than expecting the child to manage the switching independently.

For neurodivergent children, consistent sameness within your home isn't a preference—it's a neurological necessity that allows their brains to rest, regulate, and eventually build capacity to navigate inconsistency elsewhere.

# Letting Go of What You Cannot Control: Managing Your Own Distress When the Other Parent's Choices Affect Your Child

When a parent watches their child return from the other home visibly tired, emotionally dysregulated, or repeating concerning information, a particular kind of distress takes hold. It is not abstract worry—it is visceral, immediate, and often intense. The parent sees evidence that something in the other household is affecting their child's well-being, and the powerlessness of being unable to change it can feel unbearable. This distress is real, valid, and also problematic if left unmanaged, because children are exquisitely attuned to their parent's emotional state and will absorb that anxiety as information about their own safety.

Research on parental emotion regulation and child outcomes consistently demonstrates that a parent's ability to manage their own distress directly influences their child's capacity to regulate during stressful transitions. When a parent greets their returning child while internally flooded with frustration about the co-parent's choices—late bedtimes, inconsistent meals, screen time without limits—that emotional state communicates itself through facial expressions, body tension, and tone of voice even when words remain neutral. The child, already navigating the complexity of two different homes, now carries an additional burden: the sense that their presence from the other home has upset this parent, creating an impossible loyalty bind.

The work of letting go begins with distinguishing between what serves the child and what serves the parent's need for control. A parent cannot make the co-parent follow a bedtime routine, serve vegetables, limit sugar, enforce homework time, or use gentle discipline. A parent cannot prevent the co-parent from introducing new partners too quickly, speaking negatively about them, or maintaining a chaotic household.

These realities are painful, particularly when the parent has worked so hard to create stability and sees it undermined every time the child returns. But attempting to control these circumstances—through repeated confrontations, detailed co-parenting emails that go unanswered, or efforts to document every concerning choice—often escalates conflict without changing outcomes, and the child feels the tension of that ongoing battle.

What a parent can control is their own response in the moment their child walks through the door. They can notice their body's signals of distress — the tightness in their chest, the clenched jaw, the urge to immediately ask questions about what happened at the other house—and choose to pause before responding. This pause is not about dismissing legitimate concern. It is about creating enough space between the triggering information and the response that the parent can show up for their child as a regulated, steady presence rather than as another source of anxiety.

Practical regulation techniques for these moments include simple somatic practices: taking three slow breaths before the child arrives, physically shaking out tension in the arms and legs, placing a hand on the chest to ground attention in the body rather than racing thoughts. These are not elaborate self-care rituals that require time you might not have. They are small, manageable practices that interrupt the body's stress response long enough to allow the prefrontal cortex—the part of the brain responsible for thoughtful response rather than reactive emotion—to come back online.

For neurodivergent parents or those with trauma histories, this regulation work may require additional support. Parents with ADHD may benefit from external reminders—a note on the door that says "Breathe first"—to interrupt automatic reactivity. Parents with anxiety may need to externalize worries by writing them down immediately after the child's arrival, creating a boundary between the parent's processing and the child's reentry into the home.

The goal is not to stop caring about what happens in the other home. The goal is to care in a way that does not transfer the parent's distress onto the child, allowing the child to experience this home as a place where they can simply arrive, be welcomed, and rest.

The reality that many parents face—building stability for their child while the other home operates from an entirely different playbook—is one of the loneliest aspects of co-parenting after separation. It contradicts nearly every piece of advice about consistency, cooperation, and united fronts. It leaves parents wondering whether their efforts matter at all when their child returns from the other home having experienced something completely different. And it requires a fundamental shift in how parents understand what their child actually needs to feel safe.

What this chapter has worked to establish is this: your child does not need two identical homes to develop healthy regulation, secure attachment, and felt safety. Your child needs one home where the patterns hold steady, where emotions are met with calm, where they can predict what comes next and trust that you will remain grounded when they cannot. That home can be yours, and the foundation you build there will matter profoundly, even when you cannot control what happens elsewhere.

The single-home foundation you create—through predictable routines, consistent rules, and steady emotional presence—becomes something your child internalizes over time. When your seven-year-old knows that bedtime in your home always follows the same sequence, her nervous system learns to anticipate rest, regardless of what happened the night before at her other parent's house. When your five-year-old experiences the same calm response to big feelings every time he melts down after a transition, he begins to build the internal template that says some adults can be counted on to stay steady. This internalization is not immediate, and it is not always visible, but it is happening beneath the surface of daily life, shaping how your child's brain learns to navigate an unpredictable world.

The language you use to talk about differences between homes teaches your child whether they must choose sides or whether they can hold complexity without guilt. When you name differences neutrally—"At this house we do it this way, at Dad's house it's different, and both are okay"—you give your child permission to belong in both places without betraying either parent. This permission is a gift that protects them from the divided loyalties that research consistently identifies as among the most damaging aspects of divorce for young children.

For neurodivergent children who need sameness to feel safe, the scaffolding you provide within your own home—picture schedules, comfort objects, explicit verbal support—compensates for the neurological challenges of navigating inconsistency. These adaptations are not about making your child more flexible or resilient in ways their brain cannot support. They are about building external structures that allow their nervous system to rest, regulate, and develop the felt safety they need to function well.

Perhaps the most difficult work this chapter asks of parents is the work of letting go—releasing the need to control what happens in the other home, managing the distress that arises when the co-parent's choices affect the child, and choosing to focus energy on what can actually be influenced. This letting go is not resignation or indifference. It is a strategic redirection of limited emotional resources toward the place where they will make the most difference: in your own responses, in your own home, in the moments when your child is with you and needs you to be steady.

You cannot create perfect consistency across two homes. But you can create enough safety, predictability, and emotional grounding in your home so that your child develops the internal resources to navigate imperfection. That is not a compromise. That is enough.

## CHAPTER 6

# <u>The Words That Help</u>
## Co-Parenting Communication Scripts for Helping Kids Adjust to Divorce and Family Transitions

Your five-year-old asks at breakfast, "Why can't you and Daddy just be friends and live together again?" and you pause, coffee cup halfway to your mouth, aware that whatever you say next matters deeply. Later that night, your seven-year-old whispers into the dark, "Is it my fault you don't love each other anymore?" and you realize that the silence you thought was protecting her has left space for her to fill in the gaps with fears far worse than the truth.

Finding the right words to talk with kids in this age group about divorce and two homes is one of the most anxiety-provoking aspects of separation for parents. The fear of saying something wrong, of causing harm, of making promises you cannot keep, or of making things worse can leave parents feeling stuck—choosing silence or vague reassurances that leave children more confused than comforted. At the same time, children are noticing everything: the tone of your voice during phone calls with your ex, the way you stiffen when the doorbell rings for pickup, the careful way you avoid certain topics. When parents don't provide clear, honest, age-appropriate information, young children create their own explanations, and those explanations often center on themselves as the cause of their family's pain.

This chapter provides the specific language and communication scripts that help young children process the reality of living in two households without being overwhelmed by adult complexity or conflict. These are not perfect speeches delivered in ideal moments—they are real, usable phrases for the everyday questions that come up at bedtime, in the car on the way to transitions, during difficult moments, and in the quiet times when your child is trying to make sense of their changing world. The goal is not to have all the answers or to explain everything perfectly, but to offer your child clarity, reassurance, and emotional honesty that matches their developmental capacity to understand.

Children between ages three and eight think differently than adults do. They are concrete thinkers who struggle with abstract concepts like "we grew apart" or "it's complicated." They experience time differently, making it hard to understand permanence or future possibilities.

At this developmental stage, they naturally view the world from their own perspective, which means they often assume they are the center of cause and effect in their world. These developmental realities shape what children need to hear and how they can process information about divorce. A three-year-old needs different words than a seven-year-old, and an autistic child who processes language literally needs different explanations than a neurotypical peer who can grasp metaphor.

This chapter also addresses the difficult reality that you cannot control what your ex-partner says to your child about the separation, about you, or about the future. You may be working hard to provide honest, reassuring explanations while your ex-partner offers conflicting messages, blames you in front of your child, or makes promises they cannot keep. The scripts and approaches in this chapter focus on what you can say in your own home and relationship with your child—language that builds trust, validates feelings, and provides a steady emotional anchor regardless of what messages your child receives elsewhere.

For children with neurodevelopmental differences, communication about divorce benefits from additional adaptation. Children with ADHD may need shorter, more frequent conversations rather than one long explanation. Autistic children may need concrete, literal language and visual aids to understand what "two homes" actually means in their daily life. Highly sensitive children may need extra reassurance that their big feelings are normal and that you can handle their emotions without falling apart yourself.

The words you choose matter, but what matters even more is the emotional truth underneath them: that your child is safe, that the divorce is not their fault, that both parents will continue to love and care for them, and that you can hold their questions and feelings without shutting down or becoming overwhelmed. This chapter will help you find those words and deliver them with the calm, grounded presence your child needs to begin making sense of their new reality.

# What Young Children Need to Hear About Divorce: Age-Appropriate Explanations That Provide Clarity Without Adult Details (Ages 3-4, 5-6, 7-8)

Young children at different developmental stages need fundamentally different explanations about divorce because their cognitive abilities, understanding of time, and capacity to process abstract concepts change dramatically between ages three and eight. What works for a preschooler will confuse or patronize a second-grader, while explanations appropriate for older children will overwhelm and frighten younger ones. Parents often offer one explanation and assume the conversation is complete, when in reality children need repeated, evolving conversations that match their growing understanding and changing questions as they mature.

For children ages three and four, explanations must be extremely concrete and focused on immediate, tangible realities rather than abstract concepts like relationship dynamics or future possibilities. Children in this age group are still developing their understanding of cause and effect, learning to grasp permanence, and beginning to consider perspectives beyond their own immediate experience.

They need to hear that both parents love them, that they will continue to see both parents, and that nothing they did caused the separation. A three-year-old who hears "Mommy and Daddy decided to live in two different houses, but we both love you very much and you'll have a room at both homes" receives information they can actually process—concrete details about what will happen rather than abstract relationship concepts. In contrast, explanations like "we grew apart" or "we're not happy together anymore" mean nothing to a preschooler and create confusion rather than clarity.

The most critical message for this age group is that the parent who moves out has not abandoned them personally. Young children in this developmental stage often interpret a parent leaving the family home as leaving them specifically, not leaving the marriage. They need repeated reassurance delivered calmly and simply: "Daddy still loves you. Daddy will pick you up on Wednesday and you'll sleep at Daddy's house. Then you'll come back here on Friday." The concrete details about when and where matter more than explanations about why.

Children ages five and six have slightly more cognitive capacity but still think in very concrete terms and struggle with abstract relationship concepts. They can understand that parents have decided not to live together anymore, but they need clear reassurance that this decision is permanent, not something that might change if the child behaves better or wishes hard enough.

These children benefit from explanations that acknowledge the change while emphasizing continuity: "Our family is changing. Mommy and Daddy won't live in the same house anymore, but we'll both always be your parents and we'll both take care of you. You didn't cause this and you can't fix it—this is a grown-up decision."

Five- and six-year-olds often ask direct questions about whether parents still love each other, whether they might get back together, or what will happen next. Parents can answer honestly without adult details: "We care about each other, but we've decided we'll be happier living separately. This won't change. You'll have two homes now." Avoid false hope or vague possibilities that leave children waiting for reconciliation.

Children ages seven and eight can grasp more nuance and understand that relationships can end even when people aren't angry at each other, though many divorces do involve conflict these children witness. They need emotional validation of what they're observing alongside reassurance about what remains stable. An eight-year-old who has heard arguments benefits from hearing: "You know that Dad and I have been disagreeing a lot. We've decided that we'll do better living in separate homes. This doesn't change how much we both love you, and we're both still your parents forever."

Older children in this range may ask more sophisticated questions about fault, blame, or whether the divorce could have been prevented. Parents can acknowledge complexity without burdening children with adult responsibility: "Sometimes adults can't solve their problems even when they try. This is our decision, not yours. Nothing you did caused this." These children also need explicit permission to love both parents without choosing sides, especially important in high-conflict situations where loyalty pressure may be present.

## Answering the Hard Questions: Scripts for 'Why Did You Split Up?', 'Is It My Fault?', 'Will You Get Back Together?', and 'Do You Still Love Each Other?'

Children ask four questions more than any others when trying to make sense of divorce, and each question carries a specific fear that needs direct, honest addressing. These questions—"Why did you split up?", "Is it my fault?", "Will you get back together?", and "Do you still love each other?"—appear at bedtime, in the car, during transitions, and sometimes in the middle of seemingly unrelated activities when a child's mind has been working quietly on something too big to hold alone. Preparing clear, age-appropriate responses to these predictable questions helps parents provide reassurance that reduces anxiety and prevents children from creating their own, often more frightening, explanations.

**"Why did you split up?"** requires an answer that acknowledges change without burdening children with adult complexity or blame. For younger children ages three through five, the explanation needs to be simple and focused on the outcome rather than the process: "Mommy and Daddy decided we will be happier living in two different homes. This is a grown-up decision, and we both still love you very much."

For children ages six through eight who can grasp slightly more nuance, parents can add: "Sometimes grown-ups try hard to solve their problems but can't fix them. We decided this is what's best for our family." The key is to avoid details about who did what, why one parent is angry, or what specific conflicts led to the separation. Children do not need to understand the adult reasons. Instead, they need to understand that the decision is final, that it was made by both parents, and that it has nothing to do with them.

**"Is it my fault?"** must be answered immediately, firmly, and repeatedly because kids in this age group's egocentric thinking makes them assume they caused any major change in their world. The script is direct and unequivocal: "No. This is not your fault at all. Nothing you did, nothing you said, and nothing you thought caused this. This is about grown-up things between Mommy and Daddy. You are wonderful, and we both love you completely." Parents should expect to repeat this answer many times, as children will test it from different angles—asking if their behavior, their grades, their noise level, or their needs contributed to the separation. Each time, the answer remains the same: this is not about you, and you could not have prevented it.

**"Will you get back together?"** requires honesty even when it feels harsh, because false hope prolongs a child's adjustment and keeps them waiting for a reunion that will not happen. The answer must be clear: "No, we won't get back together. We've made this decision and it won't change. But we will both always be your parents, and we both love you very much." Some children will ask this question repeatedly, especially in the first year after separation, testing whether the answer might change. Consistency matters more than softening the truth, and for children who express sadness about this reality, parents can validate the feeling while maintaining the boundary: "I know you wish we could all live together again. It's okay to feel sad about that. This is still the right decision for our family."

**"Do you still love each other?"** addresses a child's confusion about how love works and whether parental love for them might also disappear. The response distinguishes between adult romantic relationships and parent-child bonds: "The love between grown-ups in a marriage is different from the love parents have for their children. Our love for you never changes and never ends. We will always be your mom and dad, and we will always love you. As husband and wife, we've decided to live separately, but as your parents, we're both here forever." This script reassures children that love is not conditional or temporary when it comes to them, even if they've witnessed their parents' romantic relationship end.

These scripts work best when delivered calmly, without defensiveness or visible distress, and when both parents offer similar messages even if they cannot coordinate directly. Children who receive consistent, honest answers to these core questions develop trust that their parents can handle hard conversations and that asking questions is safe.

## Validating Feelings Without Amplifying Anxiety: How to Acknowledge Your Child's Emotions While Providing Reassurance and Stability

When a child says "I miss Daddy" at bedtime or melts down before a transition, parents face a delicate balance: acknowledging the emotion without letting it spiral into overwhelming anxiety. The instinct to fix, minimize, or over-explain can accidentally amplify distress rather than soothe it. Young children need their feelings validated—recognized as real and acceptable— while simultaneously receiving the message that these feelings are manageable and that the parent can hold them without falling apart.

Emotional validation means naming what your child is experiencing and communicating that the emotion makes sense given the circumstances. Research shows that simply naming an emotion can significantly reduce distress in children, helping them feel understood rather than alone with overwhelming feelings. When a five-year-old says "I don't want to go to Mommy's house," a validating response sounds like: "You're feeling worried about leaving. That makes sense—transitions are hard." This acknowledges the reality of the child's experience without judgment or dismissal.

What validation does not mean is dwelling on the emotion, asking probing questions that encourage rumination, or matching the child's distress with visible parental anxiety. When a parent responds to "I miss Daddy" with "Oh sweetie, I know, it's so hard, do you miss him all the time? Does it make you so sad? Tell me everything you're feeling," they may inadvertently signal that the emotion is too big to handle, that missing the other parent is a crisis requiring extensive processing, which amplifies anxiety rather than containing it.

The key is pairing validation with reassurance and stability. After naming the emotion, parents provide an anchor: "You're feeling sad right now, and that's okay. I'm here with you, and we're going to have our special bedtime story like we always do." This combination teaches children that feelings are temporary, manageable, and do not threaten the stability of their world. The parent acts as an emotional container—present, calm, and capable of holding the child's distress without becoming overwhelmed.

For children with neurodevelopmental differences, this approach requires adaptation. Children with ADHD may need shorter validation statements followed immediately by a concrete activity that provides regulation: "You're feeling frustrated. Let's take three deep breaths together, then we'll pack your bag."

Autistic children who process language literally benefit from clear, specific validation without metaphor: "Your body feels tight and your stomach feels bad. That happens when you're nervous. You are safe, and the schedule says we leave in ten minutes."

Highly sensitive children may need extra reassurance that their big feelings are normal and that the parent can handle them: "I see you're having a lot of feelings right now. That's okay. Your feelings don't scare me, and I'm right here."

Parents cannot control what happens at the other household, and children may return with confusing messages, unprocessed emotions, or behavioral changes that reflect experiences elsewhere. In these moments, validation without interrogation matters most. A child who comes home withdrawn needs: "You seem quiet tonight. I'm here if you want to talk, and I'm here if you just want to be close." This offers connection without pressure, communicating that the parent is a safe place for whatever the child is carrying.

The goal is not to eliminate difficult emotions or prevent children from missing their other parent. The goal is to teach children that their feelings are valid, temporary, and manageable—and that expressing emotion will not overwhelm the parent or destabilize their world. This emotional scaffolding builds resilience far more effectively than attempts to fix, distract, or minimize what children are genuinely experiencing as they navigate the reality of two households.

# Communication Adaptations for Children With Neurodevelopmental Differences: Concrete Language, Visual Supports, and Processing Time for ADHD, Autistic, and Literal-Thinking Children

Neurodivergent children—including those with ADHD, autism, and literal-thinking patterns—benefit from specific communication adaptations when processing information about divorce and two-home transitions because they process language, time, and abstract concepts differently than neurotypical peers.

Standard explanations that work for many children often don't work as well for neurodivergent children, not because these children are less capable of understanding, but because they need information delivered in formats that match their processing style. Parents who adapt their communication approach can dramatically reduce anxiety and confusion for children who otherwise struggle to make sense of what divorce means in concrete, daily terms.

**Concrete language** means replacing abstract phrases with specific, literal statements that describe exactly what will happen in observable terms. When a parent tells a neurotypical six-year-old "things are going to be different now," that child might grasp the general meaning even without details. An autistic six-year-old or a child with ADHD who thinks concretely hears those words and has no idea what "different" actually means—different how, different when, different in what specific ways? The vagueness creates anxiety rather than clarity.

Instead, concrete language sounds like: "You will sleep at Mom's house on Monday, Tuesday, and Wednesday nights. You will sleep at Dad's house on Thursday, Friday, and Saturday nights. On Sunday, you'll go back to Mom's house after lunch." This tells the child exactly what will happen in terms they can visualize and understand.

Literal-thinking children, whether autistic or simply concrete processors, interpret language exactly as spoken without inferring implied meaning or metaphor. When a parent says, "we're going through a rough patch," a literal thinker does not understand this refers to relationship difficulty—they may picture an actual patch of rough ground or simply feel confused. When explaining divorce to literal thinkers, parents must avoid idioms, metaphors, and implied meanings entirely: "Dad and I have decided to live in separate houses" works better than "we've grown apart" or "we're taking some space." The first statement describes a concrete action; the second two require abstract interpretation that literal-thinking children cannot access.

Children with ADHD benefit from shorter explanations repeated multiple times rather than one long conversation, because their attention and working memory make it difficult to hold and process lengthy information. A parent might offer the same core message—"You didn't cause this, both parents love you, you'll have two homes now"—in brief conversations over several days rather than attempting to cover everything at once. This repetition is not talking down to the child; it is matching the explanation format to how ADHD brains consolidate information over time.

**Visual supports** provide external structure that helps neurodivergent children understand and remember information that would otherwise remain abstract or overwhelming. A visual calendar showing which days the child stays at which home removes the need to hold a complex schedule in working memory or to interpret verbal explanations about "every other weekend." The child can look at the calendar and see exactly where they will be.

Color-coding helps: Mom's days in blue, Dad's days in green, with small pictures of each house next to the corresponding days.

For younger children or those with more significant processing challenges, photographs of each parent's house, bedroom, and key caregivers can be attached to the calendar, so the child connects the visual schedule to actual physical places they recognize.

Social stories—short, illustrated narratives that walk through a specific situation step by step—help autistic children and anxious children prepare for transitions by showing exactly what will happen in sequence. A social story about pickup might include: "Dad will ring the doorbell. I will get my backpack. I will hug Mom goodbye. I will walk to Dad's car. We will drive to Dad's house. I will go to my room and unpack my backpack." The predictability reduces anxiety because the child knows what to expect at each step.

**Processing time** means building in pauses and silence after delivering information, resisting the urge to fill quiet space with more words or questions. Neurodivergent children often need significantly longer than neurotypical peers to process what they have heard, formulate their thoughts, and respond.

When a parent explains something about the divorce and immediately asks "do you understand?" or "how do you feel about that?", the child may not have finished processing the first piece of information yet. Instead, parents can offer information, wait quietly for thirty seconds or more, and then gently check in: "I'm going to give you some time to think about that. We can talk more later if you have questions." This respects the child's need for time to process without pressure to respond immediately.

## What to Say When You Can't Control What Your Co-Parent Says: Responding to Confusion, Conflicting Messages, and Loyalty Conflicts Without Criticism

One of the most painful realities of co-parenting is that parents cannot control what their ex-partner says to their child about the divorce, about them, or about the reasons the family separated. A child may come home repeating a version of events that feels unfair, inaccurate, or deliberately designed to undermine the other parent's relationship with the child. They may express confusion because one parent said the divorce happened for one reason while the other parent offered a completely different explanation.

They may relay messages that sound like loyalty tests: "Daddy says you're the one who wanted to split up" or "Mommy says we'd still be together if you hadn't left." These moments leave parents feeling helpless, angry, and desperate to correct the record—but responding with criticism of the ex-partner, even when that criticism feels justified, places the child directly in the middle of adult conflict and intensifies their distress rather than relieving it.

Young children cannot hold the cognitive complexity required to understand that both parents might have different perspectives on the same event, or that one parent might be offering a version of the truth that serves their own emotional needs rather than the child's understanding.

When a five-year-old hears two different explanations for why their family separated, they do not think "these are two subjective viewpoints"—they think "one of these must be wrong, and I need to figure out which one." When a seven-year-old hears one parent criticize the other, they do not separate the criticism from their own identity—they internalize that half of who they are is being rejected.

The goal when responding to conflicting messages is not to win the narrative or to ensure the child knows "the truth" as one parent sees it. The goal is to reduce the child's confusion, relieve them of the burden of choosing sides, and provide steady reassurance that they are loved and safe regardless of what different adults are saying. This requires tremendous emotional restraint, particularly when a parent feels falsely blamed or when the co-parent's version of events feels like a deliberate attack. But children are not capable of being referees, fact-checkers, or therapists for their parents' competing stories. They need at least one parent who can hold steady and refuse to pull them into the conflict.

When a child reports something the other parent said that conflicts with your explanation, the response focuses on the child's experience rather than correcting the other parent's message. A parent might say: "It sounds like you heard something different at Dad's house, and that feels confusing. Here's what I want you to know: the divorce is not your fault, both of us love you, and you don't have to choose between us or figure out who's right. Grown-ups sometimes remember things differently, and that's okay. What matters is that you're safe and loved." This script validates the confusion without requiring the child to judge which parent is telling the truth.

For children with neurodevelopmental differences who think concretely and struggle with ambiguity, conflicting messages create significant distress because they cannot reconcile two opposing statements. An autistic child or a literal-thinking child with ADHD benefits from a clear framework: "Sometimes people remember the same thing in different ways. You might remember your birthday party one way and your friend might remember it differently—both of you are telling the truth about what you remember. It's like that with grown-ups too. What stays the same is that we both love you." This offers a concrete comparison the child can understand without forcing them to choose a side.

When a child repeats a loyalty-testing statement—something clearly designed to position one parent as the good one and the other as the bad one—the response remains calm and refuses the bait. A parent might respond: "I'm glad you told me what you heard. You never have to worry about loving both of us. It's safe to love Mommy and it's safe to love Daddy. You don't have to pick." This releases the child from the impossible position of mediating adult conflict and reassures them that their love for both parents will not result in punishment or rejection.

The words parents choose when talking with young children about divorce matter deeply, but what matters even more is the emotional truth underneath those words: that the child is safe, loved, and not responsible for the family's changes.

This chapter has provided specific scripts and communication frameworks not because there is one perfect way to explain divorce, but because having specific language reduces the paralysis many parents feel when their child asks a hard question at bedtime or whispers a fear into the dark. These scripts are starting points—templates that parents can adapt to their own voice, their child's developmental stage, and the specific realities of their family situation.

Young children will ask the same questions repeatedly, testing whether the answers remain consistent and whether it is truly safe to express their confusion, sadness, or anger about living in two households. This repetition is not a sign that previous conversations failed or that the child is not listening. It reflects how young children process big information: gradually, in small pieces, returning again and again to the same core fears until they internalize reassurance through consistent, patient responses over time. Parents who understand this pattern can respond to the tenth "Is it my fault?" with the same calm clarity they brought to the first one, recognizing that each repetition is another opportunity to build trust and security.

The communication approaches in this chapter acknowledge a painful reality that many parents face: they cannot control what their ex-partner says to their child, and they may be actively working against conflicting messages, blame, or loyalty pressure coming from the other household. The strategies provided focus on what individual parents can do within their own relationship with their child—offering clear, honest information, validating feelings without amplifying anxiety, and refusing to pull children into adult conflict even when it feels desperately unfair to stay silent about the other parent's behavior.

This restraint is not about protecting an ex-partner who may not deserve protection. It is about protecting the child from the impossible burden of mediating between two competing narratives or choosing which parent to believe.

For neurodivergent children, communication about divorce requires thoughtful adaptation rather than a one-size-fits-all approach. Concrete language, visual supports, and extended time to process are not accommodations that water down the message—they are essential tools that allow ADHD, autistic, and children who think concretely to access the same reassurance and clarity that neurotypical children receive through standard explanations.

Parents who take the time to translate abstract concepts into specific, observable terms and who provide visual schedules that make "two households" concrete rather than conceptual give their neurodivergent children the gift of understanding rather than leaving them to navigate confusion alone.

The goal of these conversations is not to make divorce feel okay to children or to eliminate their sadness about family change. The goal is to provide enough clarity, honesty, and emotional safety that children can begin to make sense of their new reality without filling in the gaps with fears that are worse than the truth.

Children who receive age-appropriate information, whose feelings are validated without being amplified, and who are explicitly released from responsibility for their parents' separation develop trust that their parent can handle hard conversations. This trust becomes the foundation for ongoing communication as children grow, their understanding deepens, and new questions emerge about what divorce means for their identity, their family, and their future. Parents who start these conversations early, with honesty and compassion, build a relationship where their child knows that asking hard questions will always be met with steadiness rather than silence.

**CHAPTER 7**

# Staying Grounded When Everything Feels Overwhelming
## Emotional Regulation During High-Conflict Co-Parenting

You're standing in the driveway watching your ex-partner's car pull away with your six-year-old in the backseat, and your hands are shaking so hard you have to shove them in your pockets. The text message that came through five minutes before pickup—another criticism, another last-minute schedule change, another jab designed to unsettle you—is still burning in your mind, and you realize your daughter saw your face before you could smooth it into something calmer.

This is the reality that no one prepared you for: you're asked to be your child's steady, grounded anchor during transitions while simultaneously managing interactions with someone who may trigger every stress response in your body. You're trying to stay calm while your body's stress response is screaming danger. You're trying to model regulation while feeling anything but regulated yourself.

Here's what matters most: your child's ability to stay emotionally safe during transitions is directly connected to your ability to manage your own nervous system responses. This isn't about being perfect or never feeling overwhelmed— it's about recognizing when you're overwhelmed and having tools to return to a grounded state before, during, and after difficult moments with your co-parent. Young children, especially those who are neurodivergent or have heightened sensory awareness, are extraordinarily attuned to their parent's emotional state. They read your body language, your tone of voice, the tension in your shoulders, the tightness around your eyes. When you're flooded with stress hormones during a handoff, your child feels that in their own body, even if you're trying to hide it.

This chapter is not about adding more to your already overwhelming plate. It's not about elaborate self-care routines that require time you don't have or resources you can't access. Instead, it focuses on practical, in-the-moment regulation techniques that work in real time—tools you can use in the thirty seconds before you open the door for pickup, strategies that help you recover after a triggering text message, practices that allow you to repair with your child when you do lose your cool.

The truth is that co-parenting with someone who is high-conflict, uncooperative, or dealing with their own unresolved issues requires an extraordinary amount of emotional labor. You're managing not only your child's big feelings but also your own triggered responses to someone who may know exactly which buttons to push. You're doing the work of two parents in terms of emotional regulation—holding steady for your child while your co-parent may be creating chaos. This is exhausting, and it's important to acknowledge that reality rather than pretend it's easy.

That's what this chapter offers. What you'll find here are strategies grounded in understanding how your nervous system works and what actually helps you return to regulation when you're activated. You'll learn to recognize your own dysregulation signals—the physical sensations that tell you you're moving into fight, flight, or freeze—and interrupt those patterns before they take over. You'll discover how shared regulation works between you and your child, and why your ability to stay grounded (or return to groundedness after losing it) teaches your child more about managing difficult emotions than any words you could say.

This chapter also addresses what to do when you don't stay calm—when you snap at your child, when your frustration leaks out, when you realize afterward that your own stress affected how you showed up. Repair is possible, and modeling how to recover from dysregulation is itself a powerful teaching moment, particularly for neurodivergent children who need to see that regulation isn't about perfection but about returning to safety after being knocked off balance.

Your emotional regulation isn't self-indulgence—it's the foundation that allows everything else in this book to work.

# Recognizing Your Own Dysregulation: Physical and Emotional Signs That You're Overwhelmed and Why It Matters for Your Child

Before a parent can help a child regulate during a difficult transition, they need to recognize when their own body's stress response has moved out of the optimal zone—that zone where thinking, responding, and connecting are possible. Dysregulation doesn't always show up with obvious signs. Sometimes it creeps in quietly, showing up first in the body before the mind registers what's happening.

Dysregulation often appears first in physical sensations. Physical signs often appear before emotional awareness catches up.

A parent might notice their jaw is clenched tight enough to ache, or that their shoulders have crept up toward their ears and stayed there. Breathing becomes shallow and rapid, confined to the upper chest rather than moving deep into the belly. The heart races even when sitting still. Hands might shake, palms sweat, or a wave of heat might flush through the body. Some parents report feeling suddenly cold, or experiencing a headache that seems to come from nowhere. Stomachaches, nausea, or a tight feeling in the chest can signal that the nervous system is overwhelmed, even when the parent isn't consciously aware of feeling stressed yet.

These physical responses reflect the automatic stress response shifting into a protective state—fight, flight, or freeze. The body is preparing to respond to perceived danger, which in contentious co-parenting might be an inflammatory text message, the sound of the co-parent's car pulling into the driveway, or even just the anticipation of an upcoming exchange. For parents of neurodivergent children, this physiological response may intensify when worrying about how their child will manage the transition, creating a feedback loop where parental anxiety amplifies child dysregulation and vice versa.

Emotional and behavioral signs follow closely behind the physical ones, though sometimes they emerge simultaneously. Irritability often appears first— small annoyances that wouldn't normally register suddenly feel intolerable. A parent might snap at their child over something minor, then immediately feel guilty for the disproportionate response. Feelings of overwhelm, helplessness, or a sense of urgency can flood in, making it difficult to think clearly or access the calm, grounded responses the parent knows their child needs. Some parents describe feeling numb or disconnected, as though they're watching the handoff happen from outside their own body. Others experience racing thoughts, replaying past conflicts or catastrophizing about future ones, unable to stay present in the current moment.

Impulsivity increases when overwhelmed. A parent might fire off a reactive text to the co-parent that escalates conflict, or make a decision in the heat of emotion that they later regret. The ability to pause between stimulus and response—to choose how to react rather than simply reacting—diminishes significantly when the nervous system is in a protective state.

Why does recognizing these signs matter so profoundly for children? Young children, particularly those ages three through eight, are extraordinarily attuned to their parent's emotional state. They read stress in body language, tone of voice, facial expressions, and the overall energy a parent brings into a room. When a parent is dysregulated during a transition, the child's nervous system picks up on that distress and mirrors it, even if the parent believes they're hiding their feelings successfully. This is especially true for neurodivergent children and those with sensory processing differences, who often have heightened awareness of emotional atmospheres and process ambient stress differently.

A dysregulated parent cannot effectively co-regulate a dysregulated child. Co-regulation—the process by which a calm, grounded adult helps a child's nervous system return to safety—requires that the parent be regulated first. When both parent and child are flooded, the interaction often escalates rather than soothes, leaving everyone feeling worse and reinforcing the child's association between transitions and emotional unsafety.

Recognition is the first step. A parent who notices their jaw clenching or their thoughts spiraling has created a moment of choice—a brief window to interrupt the pattern before it fully takes over.

In-the-Moment Regulation Techniques: Practical Strategies to Use Before, During, and After High-Conflict Interactions With Your Co-Parent

Recognition alone isn't enough—it opens the door to what comes next. Once a parent recognizes their own dysregulation signals, the next step is having accessible tools to interrupt the stress response and return to a grounded state. These techniques work before anticipated difficult interactions, during real-time exchanges, and after triggering moments when recovery is needed. The key is that they must be simple enough to use when thinking clearly is already compromised.

## Before High-Conflict Interactions

The minutes before a scheduled exchange or anticipated difficult conversation offer a window to prepare the nervous system. Double-inhale exhale technique—two inhales through the nose followed by a long exhale through the mouth—activates the calming system and reduces cortisol levels more effectively than standard deep breathing.

Research from Stanford University's neuroscience department demonstrates that this pattern quickly shifts the body out of fight-or-flight mode. A parent can do this in the car before walking to the door, or while waiting for the co-parent to arrive.

Grounding techniques anchor attention in the present moment rather than allowing it to spiral into past grievances or future worries. The 5-4-3-2-1 method asks a parent to notice five things they can see, four they can touch, three they can hear, two they can smell, and one they can taste. This sensory inventory interrupts rumination and brings awareness back to the body and immediate environment.

For parents of neurodivergent children who may be managing their own ADHD or sensory sensitivities, movement-based regulation can be more effective than stillness. A brief walk around the block, stretching, or even squeezing a stress ball provides proprioceptive input that helps organize the body's stress response before a stressful interaction.

## During High-Conflict Interactions

When a conversation begins to escalate or a co-parent says something triggering, in-the-moment techniques prevent reactive responses that later require repair. The pause may be the most powerful tool available—a deliberate three-second gap between hearing something and responding to it. This brief space allows the prefrontal cortex to come back online and choose a response rather than defaulting to an automatic reaction.

Naming the emotion internally without expressing it aloud helps create distance from its intensity. A parent might silently acknowledge "I'm feeling rage right now" or "This is triggering my anxiety," which activates the brain's language centers and slightly reduces the emotional charge. This technique, supported by affect labeling research from UCLA, doesn't eliminate the feeling but makes it more manageable.

Physical anchoring keeps a parent tethered to the present when emotions threaten to flood. Pressing feet firmly into the ground, placing a hand on the chest or belly, or holding onto something solid provides sensory feedback that the body is safe even when the nervous system is signaling danger.

For exchanges happening at the doorstep with children present, brevity becomes a regulation tool. Keeping interactions to essential information — "Here's her backpack", "Pickup is at five on Sunday"—limits exposure to triggers and models businesslike boundaries for children watching.

### After High-Conflict Interactions

Recovery after a difficult interaction prevents residual stress from affecting how a parent shows up for their child in the hours that follow. The body often holds tension long after the triggering moment has passed, so physical release becomes essential. Progressive muscle relaxation, shaking out the hands and arms, or even a few minutes of vigorous movement helps discharge the stress hormones still circulating.

Bilateral stimulation—activities that engage both sides of the body rhythmically—supports nervous system integration after activation. This might look like alternating tapping on the thighs, walking, or even washing dishes with attention to the back-and-forth motion. These movements engage the same mechanisms used in EMDR therapy to process difficult experiences.

For parents who find themselves replaying the interaction obsessively, a time-bound processing window can help. Setting a timer for five minutes to journal, vent to a trusted friend, or simply sit with the feelings gives them space without allowing them to consume the rest of the day. When the timer ends, the parent consciously redirects attention to what their child needs next.

These techniques are not about achieving perfect calm—they're about returning to good enough regulation so that a parent can be present, responsive, and steady for their child even when co-parenting feels impossibly hard.

## The Co-Regulation Connection: How Your Nervous System State Directly Affects Your Child's Ability to Stay Regulated During Transitions

Children's nervous systems are not designed to regulate independently during stress—they are built to borrow regulation from the adults around them. This biological reality, grounded in attachment research and nervous system science, means that a parent's internal state during transitions directly shapes whether a child can access calm or remains trapped in distress. When a parent stands at the door for a handoff with their own body's stress response in fight-or-flight mode—heart racing, jaw clenched, thoughts spiraling—their child's body reads those signals and mirrors them, even when no words are spoken.

This process happens beneath conscious awareness. A three-year-old cannot articulate that her mother's shallow breathing and tight voice are making her feel unsafe, but her nervous system registers the mismatch between her mother's words ("Everything's fine, sweetie") and the tension radiating from her body. A seven-year-old with ADHD, who experiences emotional regulation differently due to executive function differences, becomes even more dysregulated when his father's stress floods the room during packing time. The child's system asks a fundamental question during every transition: *Is my parent safe right now?* If the answer is no, the child cannot settle, no matter how perfect the routine or how carefully chosen the words.

Research on parent-child dyads demonstrates that emotional states synchronize between caregivers and children, particularly during moments of stress. Studies published in the *Journal of Family Psychology* show that children in high-conflict divorce situations who have access to at least one consistently regulated parent demonstrate significantly better mental health outcomes and more secure attachment patterns than children whose parents are both chronically overwhelmed. The parent's calm presence activates the child's social engagement system—the part of the nervous system responsible for social connection, safety, and the ability to think clearly. Without that anchor, children default to survival responses: hyperactivity, defiance, withdrawal, or physical symptoms like stomachaches and headaches.

This shared regulation connection operates continuously, not just during obvious meltdowns. A parent scrolling through hostile text messages from their co-parent while their child plays nearby transmits that activation even without direct interaction. A parent who white-knuckles their way through a handoff, appearing outwardly composed but internally flooded, still communicates unsafety through micro-expressions, tone shifts, and body tension that young children instinctively detect. Neurodivergent children and those with sensory processing differences often have heightened awareness of these subtle cues, making them more attuned to parental stress.

The implications for transitions are profound. A parent cannot effectively support their child's regulation during a difficult handoff if they themselves are dysregulated. Shared regulation requires that the parent access their own grounded state first—not perfectly, not without effort, but enough to signal to the child's nervous system that safety is available. This is why the techniques in the previous section matter so deeply: they are not luxuries or self-care extras, but essential infrastructure that allows parents to be the steady presence their child's developing brain requires.

When both parent and child are flooded simultaneously, the interaction typically escalates rather than soothes. The child's distress triggers more parental anxiety, which amplifies the child's dysregulation, creating a feedback loop that leaves everyone feeling worse. Breaking this cycle requires that the parent interrupt their own stress response first, even briefly, to create space for the child's nervous system to begin settling.

This does not mean parents must be calm at all times or never show emotion. It means recognizing when their own activation is affecting their child and having tools to return to regulation—or at minimum, to avoid transmitting additional distress during already difficult moments. The parent's nervous system becomes the child's external regulator until the child's brain develops enough to manage stress independently, a process that extends well beyond age eight and requires thousands of repetitions of being helped back to safety by a trusted adult.

## Repair and Recovery: What to Do When You Lose Your Cool in Front of Your Child and How to Model Healthy Emotional Processing

No parent navigates contentious co-parenting without losing their cool at some point. The question is not whether it will happen, but what to do when it does—and how to transform those inevitable moments of dysregulation into opportunities to teach children something profoundly important about emotional recovery. When a parent snaps at their child during packing time, or their frustration with the co-parent leaks out in a sharp tone during a handoff, repair becomes essential not just for restoring connection but for modeling that mistakes do not equal catastrophe.

Young children, particularly those ages three through eight, do not need perfect parents. They need parents who can acknowledge when they've been overwhelmed, take responsibility without shame, and demonstrate that relationships can be repaired after rupture. Research on attachment demonstrates that the repair process itself—not the absence of conflict—builds secure attachment and emotional resilience in children.

Studies published in *Developmental Psychology* show that children who regularly witness their parents recovering from emotional dysregulation with accountability and reconnection develop stronger emotion regulation skills than children whose parents either never lose control or never acknowledge when they do.

The repair process begins the moment a parent recognizes they've lost their grounding. This might be seconds after yelling, or it might be hours later when the adrenaline has cleared enough to see the situation clearly. Timing matters, but perfection does not. A parent who waits until they've genuinely calmed down offers a more authentic repair than one who rushes through an apology while still flooded with stress hormones.

The first step is approaching the child with simplicity and honesty. For younger children ages three through five, this might sound like: "I'm sorry I yelled when we were getting your backpack ready. I was feeling frustrated, and I used a loud, scary voice. That wasn't okay. You didn't do anything wrong." For children ages six through eight, slightly more context can help: "I got overwhelmed earlier and I spoke to you in a way that wasn't kind. I was upset about something that had nothing to do with you, and I didn't manage my feelings well. I'm sorry."

What matters most is that the apology centers the child's experience rather than the parent's justification. Explanations that blame the co-parent—"I only yelled because your dad changed the schedule again"—teach children that emotional outbursts are someone else's fault and that they must manage adult conflict. Instead, the parent models ownership: "I made a choice I'm not proud of, and I'm working on doing better."

For neurodivergent children, particularly those with autism who process language literally or those with ADHD who may have internalized past criticism, the repair conversation benefits from extra clarity. A parent might add: "When I yelled, that was about my feelings, not about you. You are safe. I am working on staying calmer, and I will keep practicing." Physical reconnection—a hug, sitting close, or simply being present without pressure—helps regulate children whose body's stress responses remain activated after witnessing parental distress.

After the immediate repair, the parent demonstrates emotional processing by naming what they're doing to recover. This might look like saying aloud, "I'm going to take some deep breaths now to help my body calm down," or "I'm going to take a short walk to clear my head." These narrations teach children that emotions are manageable, that adults experience overwhelm too, and that there are tools available when feelings become too big.

Repair is not a one-time event but an ongoing practice. Each time a parent loses their cool and then returns to reconnect with honesty and warmth, they teach their child that mistakes do not break relationships—and that recovery is always possible. This lesson, repeated across childhood, becomes the foundation for how children will navigate their own emotional storms for years to come.

# Building Your Regulation Toolkit: Creating Sustainable Practices That Fit Into Real Life Without Adding to Your Overwhelm

The idea of building a regulation toolkit can feel like one more impossible task on an already overwhelming list. Parents navigating contentious co-parenting are already managing work schedules, household responsibilities, their child's emotional needs, and the constant stress of difficult interactions with an ex-partner. The thought of adding self-care practices or regulation routines can trigger immediate resistance—not because parents don't recognize their importance, but because there simply isn't space for anything else.

This is why sustainable regulation practices must be small, integrated into existing routines, and immediately accessible during moments of stress rather than requiring dedicated time that doesn't exist. The goal is not to create an elaborate self-care regimen but to identify a handful of tools that work in real time—techniques that take thirty seconds before opening the door for a handoff, strategies that fit into the three minutes between receiving a triggering text and needing to respond, practices that help a parent recover during the drive home after dropping their child off.

Research on habit formation demonstrates that sustainable behavior change happens through tiny, consistent actions rather than dramatic overhauls. A study published in the *European Journal of Social Psychology* found that simple behaviors repeated in consistent contexts become automatic in an average of sixty-six days, meaning that a parent who practices one grounding technique before every transition will eventually access that regulation response without conscious effort. The key is choosing practices that require minimal cognitive load and can be performed even when already stressed.

## Micro-Practices That Fit Into Transition Routines

The most effective regulation tools integrate into existing co-parenting routines. Before each handoff, a parent might practice double-inhale exhale technique—two quick inhales through the nose followed by a long exhale—while walking from the car to the door. This takes five seconds and immediately reduces cortisol levels. After receiving a difficult message from the co-parent, a parent might place one hand on their chest and one on their belly, feeling the rise and fall of breath for three cycles before deciding whether to respond. During the drive home after dropping off their child, a parent might name three things they can see, two they can hear, and one they can physically feel, anchoring attention in the present rather than ruminating on what just happened.

For parents of neurodivergent children who may themselves be neurodivergent with ADHD or sensory processing differences, movement-based regulation often works better than stillness. A parent might do ten jumping jacks before a stressful phone call, squeeze a stress ball during a tense conversation, or take a brief walk around the block after a difficult exchange. These practices provide proprioceptive input that helps organize the nervous system without requiring the executive function to sit quietly and meditate.

## Building a Personalized Toolkit

Not every regulation technique works for every person, and trying to force a practice that doesn't fit creates more stress rather than less. A parent's regulation toolkit should include two to three techniques that genuinely feel accessible and effective for their specific body's stress response and life circumstances. Some parents find that listening to a particular song in the car after drop-off helps them transition back to their own emotional state. Others benefit from texting a trusted friend a simple code word that means "I need support but can't talk right now." Some parents keep a small object in their pocket—a smooth stone, a piece of fabric, a meaningful token—that they can touch during difficult moments to remind themselves they are safe even when their nervous system is signaling danger.

The regulation toolkit is not about perfection or doing everything right. It is about having one or two reliable tools within reach when the hard moments come—and they will come. These small practices, repeated consistently, become the infrastructure that allows parents to stay grounded enough to be the steady presence their child needs, even when co-parenting feels impossibly hard.

Staying grounded during contentious co-parenting is not a one-time task—it is ongoing, repetitive, and often invisible labor that no one witnesses or applauds. A parent who pauses for three seconds before responding to a triggering text, who practices grounding breaths in the driveway before a handoff, who repairs with their child after losing their cool—that parent is doing profound work that directly protects their child's emotional safety during one of the most stressful experiences of childhood.

This chapter has focused on a truth that bears repeating: a parent cannot effectively support their child's regulation during transitions if they themselves are chronically overwhelmed. The co-regulation connection between parent and child means that the parent's nervous system state becomes the child's external regulator, particularly for young children ages three through eight whose brains are not yet capable of managing big emotions independently. When a parent recognizes their own dysregulation signals—the clenched jaw, the racing heart, the spiraling thoughts—and uses accessible tools to return to groundedness, they are not engaging in self-indulgence. They are building the essential infrastructure that allows them to be the steady, safe presence their child needs.

The techniques offered in this chapter are intentionally simple because they must work in real time, during moments when thinking clearly is already compromised. Double-inhale exhale technique before a difficult interaction, grounding through sensory awareness during a tense exchange, physical movement to discharge stress afterward—these practices take seconds, not hours, and fit into the reality of daily life rather than requiring dedicated time that overwhelmed parents do not have. For neurodivergent parents or those managing ADHD, sensory processing differences, or executive function variations who are raising neurodivergent children, movement-based and sensory-focused regulation tools often prove more accessible than traditional mindfulness practices that require sustained attention and stillness.

The repair process after losing control teaches children something equally important: that mistakes do not break relationships, that adults experience overwhelm too, and that recovery is always possible. When a parent approaches their child with honest accountability—"I'm sorry I yelled. I was feeling frustrated and I didn't manage my feelings well. You didn't do anything wrong"—they model emotional processing that will shape how that child navigates their own difficult feelings for years to come. This is particularly important for neurodivergent children who may have experienced repeated criticism or correction and benefit from clear reassurance that parental dysregulation is not their fault or responsibility to fix.

Building a sustainable regulation toolkit is not about adding more tasks to an already overwhelming schedule. It is about identifying two or three techniques that genuinely work for a parent's specific nervous system and life circumstances, then practicing them consistently in the contexts where they're needed most. These micro-practices, repeated across weeks and months, become automatic responses that help parents interrupt stress cycles before they fully take over.

The reality remains that co-parenting with someone who is high-conflict, uncooperative, or dealing with unresolved issues requires extraordinary emotional labor. Parents doing this work are managing not only their child's big feelings but also their own triggered responses to someone who may deliberately provoke distress. This chapter validates that difficulty while offering hope: even when a parent cannot control their co-parent's behavior, they can learn to manage their own nervous system responses in ways that shield their child from adult conflict and model resilience through adversity. That work, done imperfectly but consistently, is enough.

CHAPTER 8

# Building Belonging Across Two Homes
## Long-Term Emotional Support and Resilience for Young Children Through Separation

Your eight-year-old daughter casually mentions "my room at Dad's" while drawing at your kitchen table, and something in your chest both lifts and aches—she's found a way to hold each household as hers. It's been two years since the separation, and you're starting to see something you couldn't have imagined in those early, terrible months: she's not just surviving the back-and-forth anymore, she's building a life that includes both places, both parents, without constantly looking over her shoulder to see if that's allowed.

This chapter is about that longer journey—the one that extends beyond managing this week's handoff or getting through tonight's bedtime. It's about how young children, over time, develop genuine belonging across two homes rather than simply learning to cope with transitions. Belonging is different from adjustment. Adjustment means your child has stopped crying at drop off. Belonging means your child has internalized that each household are real places where they are loved, known, and safe—that their life isn't split in half but rather held in two places at once.

For children ages three through eight, what belonging looks like changes dramatically as they grow. A four-year-old's sense of home is tied to physical objects, familiar smells, and the presence of their parent. By seven or eight, children begin to develop a more complex understanding of identity and place—they can hold the idea that home isn't just one location, that love doesn't divide when it's shared across households. This developmental progression matters because the strategies that build belonging for a preschooler differ from what an early elementary child needs, and parents benefit from understanding where their child is in this journey.

The work of building belonging happens slowly, through hundreds of small moments rather than through any single conversation or intervention. It happens when you consistently welcome your child back from the other home without interrogation or criticism. It happens when you help your five-year-old pack his favorite stuffed animal to take to Dad's house, communicating through your actions that it's safe to love both places. It happens when you validate your seven-year-old's excitement about the new puppy at Mom's house, even when it stings that you weren't part of that decision.

For neurodivergent children—including those with ADHD, autism, dyslexia, or high sensitivity—building belonging presents unique challenges. These children often need more sameness, more predictability, and more sensory comfort to feel regulated and secure. When those needs aren't met equally in both households, or when one parent doesn't understand or accommodate their neurodivergent profile, these children may struggle to feel genuinely at home in both places. This chapter addresses how to support your neurologically different child's sense of belonging within what you can control, while acknowledging the reality that you cannot force the other household to provide the same level of understanding or accommodation.

This chapter also teaches you to recognize the difference between a child who is truly thriving and one who has learned to perform okayness to protect their parents' feelings. Young children are remarkably skilled at reading what adults need from them, and sometimes what looks like successful adjustment is actually a child suppressing their real feelings to avoid causing conflict. You'll learn what genuine resilience looks like at different ages and how to create the conditions within your own home and relationship that allow your child to be honest about their experience rather than performing happiness.

Here's what I've learned to be true: you cannot control whether your child feels belonging at their other home. You cannot force your co-parent to create emotional safety or meet your child's developmental needs. What you can do is build something steady, warm, and genuine in your own home—a foundation of belonging that contributes to your child's overall sense of being held and loved as they grow, regardless of what happens elsewhere.

# What Belonging Means to Young Children at Different Ages: Moving Beyond Adjustment to Genuine Security and Identity Across Two Homes (Ages 3-4, 5-6, 7-8)

Understanding what belonging means to your child requires recognizing that it changes fundamentally as they develop. A three-year-old's sense of home lives in their body and in the immediate present moment, while an eight-year-old is beginning to construct a more abstract understanding of identity that can hold complexity. These differences matter because the strategies that help a preschooler feel secure won't necessarily translate to what an older child needs as they grow into a more sophisticated understanding of their family structure.

For children ages three and four, belonging is almost entirely sensory and relational. At this developmental stage, home is where their special blanket lives, where they know the smell of the kitchen in the morning, where their parent's voice sounds when calling them to dinner. At this age, belonging means emotional attunement—the felt sense that their parent notices when they're upset, responds when they're scared, and provides comfort when the world feels too big.

These young children experience belonging through mutual regulation, the process of calming down in the presence of a steady adult whose nervous system helps settle theirs. When a three-year-old returns from the other home and melts into your arms, they're not manipulating or being dramatic — they're seeking the mutual regulation that tells their body they belong here, they're safe, you're attuned to them.

What researchers have found—and what I've seen play out in countless families—is that children this age build security through consistent, responsive caregiving that helps them internalize the capacity to self-soothe over time. For neurodivergent children, particularly those with autism or differences in how they process sensory input, belonging at this age may depend even more heavily on specific sensory anchors—the same cup for water, the same bedtime song, the same texture of pajamas—because these concrete elements provide the predictability their nervous systems require to feel safe.

As children reach ages five and six, their understanding of belonging begins to shift—they can now grasp it as something that extends beyond the immediate moment. They can hold the idea of "my room at Mom's" and "my room at Dad's" without those concepts canceling each other out, though this understanding is still fragile and needs reinforcement. At this stage, belonging means acceptance—the feeling that each household welcome them fully, that they don't have to hide parts of themselves or their experience to fit in either place.

Five- and six-year-olds are also beginning to internalize family routines as part of their identity, which is why consistency in daily rhythms matters so much. When bedtime looks similar in each household, when both parents use similar language to talk about feelings, children this age experience less cognitive dissonance and more integrated belonging. They're also acutely sensitive to feeling torn between parents, watching carefully to see if mentioning one parent upsets the other. Children with ADHD may struggle particularly at this age with the planning and organization skills demands of tracking two different sets of rules or expectations, which can undermine their sense of belonging if they're constantly "getting it wrong" in one home or the other.

As children reach ages seven and eight, they develop a more complex, identity-based understanding of belonging. They're beginning to see themselves as part of multiple communities—family, school, neighborhood—and can hold the reality that family can look different from their friends' families while still being valid and whole. At this age, belonging means having agency in their own story.

These older children benefit from being included in age-appropriate conversations about schedules and transitions, from having their preferences heard even when they can't always be accommodated, from understanding that their feelings about the divorce and the two-home arrangement are allowed to be complicated.

Research on middle childhood development shows that children this age are constructing their self-concept through relationships and social contexts, which means they're actively working to integrate their two-home experience into a coherent sense of who they are. For neurodivergent children, particularly those who are autistic and think concretely, this age brings the challenge of reconciling two different environments that may have vastly different sensory profiles, social expectations, or communication styles—belonging requires support in holding that complexity without feeling fragmented.

## The Long View of Resilience: How Consistent Emotional Support Over Time Builds Internal Security Rather Than Just Coping Skills

Resilience is often misunderstood as a child's ability to bounce back quickly from difficulty, to stop crying faster, to appear unaffected by hard things. But true resilience—the kind that serves children throughout their lives—is not about developing a thick skin or learning to suppress distress.

It is about building emotional security, a deep-down sense that they are loved, that the world is fundamentally safe enough, and that they have the capacity to manage difficult feelings when they arise. This kind of resilience develops slowly, over years, through the accumulation of thousands of small moments in which a parent shows up consistently, responds with warmth, and provides emotional safety even when everything else feels uncertain.

For young children navigating life between two homes, the difference between coping skills and internal security matters enormously. Coping skills are strategies children use to get through hard moments—distraction techniques, breathing exercises, transition objects that comfort them during handoffs. These tools have value, particularly in acute moments of distress, and this book has offered many such strategies throughout previous chapters. But coping skills alone do not build the foundation children need for long-term emotional health. A child can learn to take deep breaths during transitions while still carrying a fundamental anxiety about whether they truly belong in both homes, whether their parents will remain stable, whether expressing their real feelings will cause the adults they love to fall apart.

Internal security, by contrast, is what happens when consistent emotional support over time teaches a child's nervous system that they are safe, that their feelings are manageable, and that their parents can handle their distress without becoming overwhelmed or withdrawn.

Research on attachment and child development demonstrates that children develop this internal security through repeated experiences of emotional responsiveness—moments when their emotional signals are noticed, understood, and responded to with care.

When a four-year-old melts down at bedtime on transition nights and their parent consistently responds with calm presence rather than frustration, that child begins to internalize the message that big feelings are not dangerous, that they will not be abandoned when they struggle, that they are worthy of patience and care. Over months and years, these repeated experiences build what developmental psychologists call an "internal working model"—a template for how relationships work and how worthy the child is of love and support.

This process cannot be rushed. A parent cannot create internal security through a single perfect conversation or one well-executed transition. It develops through the steady accumulation of repair after conflict, of reassurance after fear, of presence during distress. It develops when a parent welcomes their six-year-old home from the other household with the same warmth every single time, regardless of how the exchange with the co-parent went. It develops when a seven-year-old asks the same worried question for the twentieth time—"Will you still be here when I get back?"—and receives the same patient, honest answer they received the previous nineteen times.

For neurologically different children, building internal security requires additional scaffolding because their nervous systems may be more easily emotionally overwhelmed and slower to return to baseline.

An autistic child who experiences transitions as sensory and emotional overwhelm needs not just coping strategies for the moment but also the repeated experience of a parent who understands their specific needs, who doesn't shame their meltdowns, who provides the same sensory comforts and predictable routines every time they return home. A child with ADHD who struggles with emotional regulation needs a parent who can stay calm through their intensity, who doesn't interpret their big reactions as manipulation, who offers mutual regulation consistently enough that the child begins to internalize those calming strategies as their own capacity.

The long view of resilience means trusting that what you do today—the calm you bring to this transition, the validation you offer after that meltdown, the steady routine you maintain despite your exhaustion—is building something in your child that will serve them long after they've grown beyond needing your hand to hold during handoffs.

## Recognizing Thriving Versus Compliance: Signs Your Child Is Genuinely Building Belonging Rather Than Just Performing Okayness

One of the most difficult distinctions for parents to make is recognizing whether their child is genuinely thriving in the two-home arrangement or simply performing okayness to protect the adults around them. Young children are remarkably skilled at reading what their parents need from them, and sometimes what looks like successful adjustment is actually a child who has learned to suppress their real feelings to avoid causing conflict or adding to a parent's visible distress. Understanding the difference matters because compliance masquerading as resilience can lead to internalized anxiety, emotional suppression, and long-term difficulties with authentic self-expression.

Genuine thriving in children ages three through eight shows up in their spontaneous behavior, not in their carefully managed responses to direct questions. A child who is building real belonging across two homes will often mention both parents and both households naturally in conversation without monitoring the listener's reaction first.

A six-year-old who says at breakfast, "Dad and I saw a really cool truck yesterday," without first checking your face for signs of hurt or anger is demonstrating that she feels safe loving both parents openly. She is not performing neutrality or hiding her affection for her other parent to protect your feelings. What we know from research on child development and family transitions is that children who feel secure across multiple caregiving environments show this kind of unguarded emotional expression, freely sharing experiences from both homes without loyalty conflict or self-censorship.

Children who are thriving also show relatively quick emotional regulation after transitions. While it is entirely normal for young children to need some time to settle in after a handoff—particularly neurologically different children who require longer processing periods—a child who is building genuine belonging will typically relax within a reasonable timeframe and reengage with their environment. A seven-year-old who walks in the door, takes off his shoes, and starts telling you about his weekend within twenty minutes is showing signs of secure attachment and comfort in your home.

By contrast, a child who remains emotionally flat for hours, who avoids eye contact, who goes straight to his room and stays there, or who seems to be performing cheerfulness with a brittle quality may be signaling that something is not right—that he is managing adult emotions rather than processing his own.

Compliance often appears as emotional caretaking. When a four-year-old pats her mother's arm and says, "It's okay, Mommy, don't be sad," she is not demonstrating resilience—she is taking on the role of comforter, reversing the parent-child dynamic in a way that undermines her own sense of security. Similarly, when an eight-year-old carefully avoids mentioning his father because he has learned that doing so upsets his mother, he is not thriving—he is performing emotional labor to maintain peace.

What research on parentification and role reversal tells us is that these patterns, while they may look like maturity or kindness, actually increase anxiety and interfere with healthy emotional development because the child is prioritizing the parent's emotional state over their own authentic experience.

Another key indicator is how children respond to open-ended questions about their feelings. A child who is genuinely building belonging will offer varied, honest emotional responses over time—sometimes happy, sometimes frustrated, sometimes confused. A child who is performing okayness will consistently respond with surface-level reassurances: "I'm fine," "It's good," "Everything's okay." This kind of emotional flattening, particularly when paired with a child's vigilance about parental reactions, suggests that the child has learned it is safer to hide their real feelings than to risk upsetting the adults they depend on.

For neurologically different children, compliance may look different. An autistic child might script phrases they have learned are expected—"I had a good time at Mom's"—without genuine emotional connection to the words. A child with ADHD might perform hyperactive cheerfulness to mask underlying dysregulation. Recognizing these patterns requires parents to look beyond surface behavior to the quality of emotional presence underneath.

## Supporting Identity Development for Neurodivergent Children: Helping ADHD, Autistic, and Highly Sensitive Children Build Belonging When Their Needs Aren't Met Equally in Both Homes

When a neurodivergent child's needs are understood and accommodated in one home but not the other, the impact extends far beyond daily frustration—it affects their developing sense of self, their understanding of whether they are fundamentally acceptable as they are, and their capacity to build genuine belonging across both households.

A seven-year-old autistic child who has a predictable sensory-friendly space, visual schedules, and patient processing time at Mom's house but faces constant criticism for being "too slow" or "too rigid" at Dad's house is not simply dealing with inconsistent parenting—she is receiving fundamentally different messages about whether her neurodivergent brain is something to accommodate or something to fix.

Over time, this disparity can fragment her sense of identity, teaching her that she must mask or suppress core parts of herself to be accepted in one environment while being allowed to exist more authentically in the other.

What research on neurodivergent children and family transitions shows us is that routine, predictability, and sensory consistency are not preferences but neurological requirements for emotional regulation and secure attachment. When these elements are disrupted through transitions between households that operate with vastly different levels of understanding, neurodivergent children experience heightened dysregulation, increased anxiety, and difficulty developing the emotional security that comes from feeling consistently understood.

For children with ADHD, inconsistent expectations around planning and organization skills tasks—packing, transitions, remembering routines—can lead to persistent feelings of inadequacy when one home provides scaffolding and the other expects independent management beyond the child's developmental capacity. For highly sensitive children, the sensory and emotional overwhelm of moving between a calm, regulated household and a chaotic or overstimulating one can create a constant state of nervous system activation that undermines their ability to feel at home in either place.

The challenge for parents is that you cannot control what happens in your co-parent's household. You cannot force them to understand your child's neurodivergent profile, to read the books you've shared, to implement the strategies the therapist recommends, or to stop interpreting sensory meltdowns as manipulation.

What you can control is building something steady and affirming within your own home—a foundation of belonging that validates your child's neurologically different experience and provides the accommodations their nervous system requires to feel safe, even when the other household does not offer the same understanding.

This means creating an environment where your child's neurodivergent traits are not problems to be solved but differences to be honored. For an autistic child, this might mean maintaining the same morning routine every single day they are with you, using visual schedules that reduce anxiety about what comes next, and never rushing them through transitions even when you are running late.

For a child with ADHD, it might mean breaking down the overwhelming task of packing for the other home into tiny, manageable steps with visual checklists, offering body-based regulation tools like fidgets or movement breaks, and responding to their emotional intensity with calm presence rather than frustration.

For a highly sensitive child, it might mean creating a sensory-safe space in your home where they can decompress after the overstimulation of transitions, honoring their need for quiet and downtime, and validating their big feelings without trying to talk them out of their emotional reality.

You also support your neurodivergent child's identity development by naming their experience with language that builds self-understanding rather than shame. When your six-year-old with ADHD melts down because packing feels impossible, you might say, "Your brain works really hard on lots of things at once, and sometimes that makes it tricky to know where to start. Let's do this together."

When your eight-year-old autistic child struggles with the unpredictability of the other home, you might offer, "I know it's hard when things feel different than you expected. Your brain likes to know what's coming, and that makes sense."

This kind of affirming language helps children begin to understand themselves as neurodivergent rather than broken, building the foundation for self-advocacy and self-acceptance that will serve them throughout their lives.

## Practices That Cultivate Belonging Over Time: Rituals, Conversations, and Emotional Anchors That Help Children Internalize Security as They Grow

Belonging is not built through grand gestures or perfect parenting moments. It accumulates slowly, through the steady repetition of small practices that communicate safety, predictability, and unconditional acceptance. For young children navigating life between two homes, these practices—rituals, conversations, and emotional anchors—become the infrastructure upon which they build their sense of security over time. What matters is not that every interaction is flawless, but that certain reliable patterns exist consistently enough for children to internalize them as truths about their world: I am loved here. I belong here. I will be okay.

Rituals serve as one of the most powerful tools for cultivating belonging because they create predictable moments that children can count on regardless of what else feels uncertain. These do not need to be elaborate. A ritual might be as simple as the same goodbye routine every time your child leaves for the other home—three hugs, a specific phrase you always say, a wave from the window as they walk to the car.

It might be the way you always greet them when they return: the same warm tone, the same question about what they want for dinner, the same invitation to settle in without pressure to perform happiness or immediately recount their time away. What research on attachment and family transitions shows is that these repeated, predictable interactions help children develop secure internal working models—the deep-down sense that their parent will show up in consistent, trustworthy ways even when external circumstances change.

For neurodivergent children, rituals carry additional weight because they provide the sameness and predictability their nervous systems require to feel regulated. An autistic child benefits enormously from knowing that bedtime will follow the exact same sequence every night they are with you—same order of tasks, same songs, same goodnight phrases. A child with ADHD may rely on a visual checklist ritual for packing their bag, the same steps in the same order every time, reducing the executive function overwhelm that can trigger meltdowns. These rituals are not rigidity for its own sake—they are scaffolding that allows neurodivergent children to navigate transitions without constant cognitive and emotional labor.

Conversations that cultivate belonging are those that validate your child's experience without requiring them to choose sides or manage your emotions. When your five-year-old mentions something fun that happened at Dad's house, responding with genuine warmth—"That sounds really cool, I'm glad you had fun"—communicates that it is safe to love both homes, that you can hold their joy without feeling threatened by it.

When your seven-year-old asks a hard question—"Do you still love Dad?" or "Why can't we all live together?"—answering honestly and simply without burdening them with adult details builds trust over time. Scripts like "Dad and I don't live together anymore, but we both love you completely and that will never change" offer clarity without complexity, reassurance without false promises.

These conversations also include the ones you have with yourself in your child's presence—the tone you use when mentioning the other parent, the way you handle frustration during difficult handoffs, the emotional steadiness you model when things don't go as planned. Children internalize security not just from what parents say directly to them, but from what they observe about how their parents manage stress, disappointment, and conflict.

Emotional anchors are the specific, reliable elements within your home that signal to your child that this place is theirs. This might be their special spot on the couch, the drawer that holds their favorite things, the way their room smells the same every time they return. For highly sensitive children, sensory anchors matter deeply—the softness of a particular blanket, the dimness of the nightlight, the quiet of the morning routine. These anchors communicate belonging through the body, through felt experience, in ways that transcend language and logic. Over months and years, these practices weave together into something larger than any single moment—a foundation of security that children carry with them as they grow, internalized evidence that they are held, known, and safe across both homes.

Building belonging across two homes is not a destination your child reaches and then remains at forever. It is a developmental process that unfolds over years, shifting and deepening as your child grows from preschool through early elementary school and beyond. What belonging looked like when your four-year-old needed their special blanket and your physical presence to feel safe will transform into something different by the time they are eight and beginning to understand their family structure as part of their identity. This evolution is normal, expected, and requires parents to remain attuned to where their child is developmentally rather than where they wish their child would be or where other children seem to be in their adjustment.

The work of this chapter—and of this entire book—has been to help you see your child's experience of living between two homes through their eyes first, before moving to strategy or solution.

When you understand that your five-year-old's resistance to packing is not defiance, but executive function overwhelm, when you recognize that your seven-year-old's silence after transitions is not adjustment but emotional caretaking, when you see that your autistic child's need for the same bedtime routine is not rigidity but neurological regulation, you can respond in ways that build genuine security rather than simply managing surface behavior. This understanding matters more than any single technique or script because it allows you to adapt your approach as your child grows and their needs change.

You cannot control what happens in your co-parent's household. You cannot force them to understand your child's neurodivergent profile, to maintain consistent routines, to speak about you with respect, or to prioritize your child's emotional needs over their own agenda. This reality is painful, and I think it's important to name it honestly rather than pretending that positive thinking or better communication on your part will transform an uncooperative or high-conflict co-parent into a collaborative partner.

What you can control is what you build within your own home and your own relationship with your child—the steady rituals, the validating conversations, the sensory anchors, the emotional responsiveness that communicates belonging through presence rather than perfection.

The practices offered throughout this chapter are not quick fixes. They will not eliminate your child's struggles with transitions, will not make the other household suddenly meet your child's needs, and will not erase the grief and complexity inherent in living between two homes. What they will do, over time, is build internal security—the deep-down sense your child develops that they are loved, that they belong, that they can manage difficult feelings because you have shown them, again and again, that you can hold those feelings with them without falling apart.

For neurodivergent children, this process requires additional patience, additional scaffolding, and additional grace for the reality that their path toward belonging may look different and take longer than neurotypical timelines suggest. An autistic child may need years of the same predictable routine before they internalize security. A child with ADHD may continue to need transition support well into elementary school, requiring ongoing executive function scaffolding as part of their developmental profile. A highly sensitive child may always need more processing time, more sensory comfort, and more emotional validation as part of their temperament. None of this represents failure—not yours, not theirs. It's about honoring who your child actually is rather than who you imagined they would be.

The long view of resilience means trusting that what you are doing now—the calm you bring to this week's handoff, the ritual you maintain despite your exhaustion, the way you welcome your child home with the same warmth every single time—is building something that will serve them long after they have grown beyond needing your hand to hold during transitions. You are teaching them that they are worthy of patience, that their feelings matter, that home is not a single place but a feeling of being known and held. That's belonging. And it is enough.

# CONCLUSION

Guiding a young child through the reality of living in two homes doesn't come with a perfect script or foolproof routine. There's no preparation that will make transitions feel effortless for a four-year-old who doesn't yet understand why her family looks different now. What you can offer instead is something more real and sustainable: the possibility of being good enough, steady enough, and present enough to help your child build genuine security even when their world has changed in ways they didn't choose.

Throughout this book, we've focused on what transitions feel like from your child's perspective—not because understanding their experience solves every problem, but because it changes how you show up in the moments that matter most.

When you recognize that your six-year-old's meltdown before pickup isn't defiance but communication about an internal state they can't yet name, you respond differently.

Your autistic child's firm insistence on the same goodbye routine isn't stubbornness but a neurological need for predictability in an unpredictable situation—understanding this helps you protect that routine instead of dismissing it.

And when you see that your eight-year-old's quiet compliance might be hiding internalized distress rather than indicating they're fine, you create space for their real feelings to surface safely.

The questions that brought you here—why transitions are so hard, what your child is really experiencing, how to support them when your co-parent won't cooperate, what helps neurodivergent children cope with change—don't have simple answers because the situations themselves are complex. But one thing remains consistent: your child needs you to be the steady one, the parent who stays regulated when they can't, who maintains predictability in your home even when the other household operates differently, who offers honest reassurance without making promises you can't keep.

You've learned that while you cannot control what happens in your co-parent's home, you can build a foundation of safety, routine, and emotional attunement in your own. You've also learned something crucial: supporting your child's regulation begins with managing your own nervous system.

The calm you model during difficult handoffs teaches your child more about resilience than any words you could say. You've also gained practical tools — communication scripts, transition routines, regulation strategies, observation frameworks—that work in real situations with real children who have big feelings about circumstances they didn't create.

If you're parenting a neurodivergent child, you've learned that your child's ADHD, autism, sensory sensitivities, or high sensitivity aren't barriers to adjustment but essential information about what they need to feel safe. The extra scaffolding, the visual schedules, the sensory supports, the extended processing time—these aren't just accommodations that make things easier. They're necessary supports that make things accessible.

The long-term impact of divorce on your child won't be determined by whether transitions always go smoothly or whether both homes operate identically. It will be shaped by whether they consistently experience at least one parent who sees them clearly, responds to their needs with steadiness, and helps them make sense of their feelings without shame or pressure to perform okayness they don't feel.

Here's what matters most: you don't need to be perfect. Your child doesn't need you to have all the answers or to never feel overwhelmed by the weight of doing this alone. They need you to keep showing up and keep noticing. They need you to keep offering the reassurance that both homes are real, that their feelings make sense, and that they are loved completely even when their family looks different than it used to. That is enough—you are enough.

# GLOSSARY

**Attachment:** The emotional bond between a child and caregiver that provides safety, comfort, and a secure base for exploration.

**Co-Regulation:** The process by which a calm adult helps a child regulate their emotions and nervous system through presence, tone, and connection.

**Dysregulation:** A state in which a child's emotions or behavior feel out of control because their nervous system is overwhelmed.

**Executive Function:** Mental skills that help with planning, organizing, shifting attention, remembering instructions, and managing impulses.

**Internalized Anxiety:** Anxiety that does not always show outwardly but may appear as withdrawal, perfectionism, stomachaches, or sleep difficulties.

**Loyalty Conflict:** Emotional tension a child may feel when they believe loving one parent might hurt or betray the other.

**Nervous System Response:** The body's automatic reaction to stress or safety, which can influence behavior, mood, and regulation.

**Regulation:** The ability to manage emotions, impulses, and reactions in a flexible and balanced way.

**Sensory Processing:** How the brain receives and interprets sensory input such as sound, light, touch, and movement.

**Transition Stress:** Emotional or physical strain that occurs when moving between environments, routines, or caregivers.

These terms are offered as gentle guides, not labels. They help name what children may be experiencing beneath the surface during times of change. Understanding this language can make it easier to respond with steadiness and care.

# WORKS CONSULTED

American Academy of Child and Adolescent Psychiatry. *Outbursts, Irritability & Emotional Dysregulation Resource Center.* 2022.

Bonnell, Karen, with Kristin Little. *The Co-Parenting Handbook: Raising Well-Adjusted and Resilient Kids from Little Ones to Young Adults Through Divorce or Separation.* Sasquatch Books, 2017.

Brosi, Melissa, Montoya, Brenda, and Masri, Karla. *Helping Children of Divorce Understand Their Feelings.* Oklahoma State University Extension, 2019.

Droit-Volet, Sylvie. "Children and Time." *The Psychologist,* British Psychological Society, 2012.

Lippman, Jessica G., and Paddy Greenwall Lewis. *Divorcing with Children: Expert Answers to Tough Questions from Parents and Children.* Praeger, 2008.

Moran, John A., Tyler Sullivan, and Matthew Sullivan. *Overcoming the Co-Parenting Trap: Essential Parenting Skills When a Child Resists a Parent.* 2015.

National Center for Biotechnology Information. Peer-reviewed Research Articles on Child Development, Emotional Regulation, and Stress Response (PMC database).

Ricci, Isolina. *Mom's House, Dad's House.* Touchstone, 2013.

Ricci, Isolina. *The CoParenting Toolkit.* 2015.

]University of Missouri Extension. *Helping Preschoolers and Elementary-Age Children Adjust to Divorce.* 2016.

Oklahoma State University Extension. Research publications on child emotional adjustment during divorce.

# FURTHER READING

For parents who would like to explore child development, emotional regulation, and co-parenting in greater depth:

Bonnell, Karen. *The Co-Parenting Handbook.*
Ricci, Isolina. *Mom's House, Dad's House.*
Lippman, Jessica G., and Paddy Greenwall Lewis. *Divorcing with Children.*
American Academy of Child and Adolescent Psychiatry. Resources for Families Navigating Emotional and Behavioral Challenges.

University Extension Publications on Helping Children Adjust to Divorce.

# ABOUT THE AUTHOR

**Laura Bennett, M.Ed.**

Laura Bennett is an educator and writer who supports parents navigating family change with a focus on the emotional well-being of young children ages three to eight. She holds a master's degree in education and has spent years working closely with children impacted by divorce, trauma, foster care, parental absence, and learning differences such as ADHD, autism, and dyslexia.

Known for her empathic, observant approach, Laura writes with careful attention to what young children feel but may not yet be able to say. Her work helps parents respond to emotional signals expressed through behavior, play, routine disruption, and regulation challenges with steadiness, clarity, and care that foster safety, trust, and resilience.

Laura writes practical, compassionate nonfiction for parents who want to move through divorce and family change without asking their children to carry adult pain. Her work offers developmentally informed insight, steady reassurance, and tools grounded in both professional experience and deep listening.

# MORE FROM
# THE STEADY GROUND SERIES

The *Steady Ground Series* is designed to support parents and young children through life's most tender and uncertain transitions. Each book offers calm guidance, developmentally sensitive language, and reassurance that emotional security can remain steady - even when family circumstances change.

If this book has been helpful to you, other titles in the series may offer additional clarity, comfort, and practical support as your family continues to grow and adapt.

## Available titles

### Talking to Young Children Ages 3–8 About Divorce and Parental Addiction: Answering the Hard Questions with Compassion and Clarity

A compassionate guide to helping young children understand family change while preserving emotional safety and trust.

### Helping Young Children Ages 3–8 Navigate Life Between Two Homes: Answering the Hard Questions With Compassion and Clarity

A gentle guide to helping young children build stability, trust, and emotional security while living between two homes.